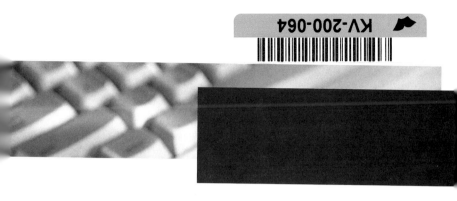

Preface

This third edition of the *Internet Resource Guide for Nurses and Health Care Professionals* has been updated and expanded to reflect the rapidly changing issues and trends seen in relation to the Internet. The book provides background information about the Internet, services that it provides, and various types of Internet resources available for nursing and health care professionals and students. Our goal is that, after reading this book, you will have the knowledge and confidence you need to use the Internet effectively. The Internet is a tool that facilitates professional networking and disseminates health care information and education to professionals and consumers. A brief description of each chapter follows.

The first chapter defines the Internet and summarizes the benefits that online resources offer the health care professional and consumer. This chapter also lists requirements for Internet access and criteria to help you select an Internet service provider.

Chapter 2 describes services available on the Internet, emphasizing electronic mail and how to find particular topics on the World Wide Web. This chapter includes current information on instant messaging. Special features of this chapter include a section on Web search strategies and information on listservs, news groups, and other Web resources.

Chapter 3 provides guidelines for "netiquette" and evaluating information found on the Web; it also addresses Internet security issues.

Chapter 4 discusses factors that make online learning attractive. It also describes the educational opportunities that can be found on the Internet, ranging from informal learning to degree programs. Special features include the following:

- How various online services and resources facilitate learning.

- Points for students to consider prior to enrolling in distance learning or Web-based programs.

- Criteria for the evaluation of instructional Web sites.

Chapter 5 addresses research on the Internet, exploring some of the many ways that formal and informal research can be facilitated using the Internet, including the identification of topics for study via discussion groups, online literature and Web searches, online administration of questionnaires, collaboration with peers via e-mail, learning about funding opportunities, and the rapid dissemination of research findings via online publications.

Chapter 6 discusses using the Internet to explore career resources and opportunities.

The seventh and final chapter lists a number of Web sites and other online resources that are of particular interest to nurses and other health care professionals. These sites are organized by general categories, including career resources, professional organizations and associations, accrediting bodies, educational sites, government agencies, health care informatics, and sites for online publications. A list of frequently asked questions is included in Appendix A. Appendix B provides exercises and Appendix C provides steps for creating a personal Web page. A glossary is included to acquaint the reader with unfamiliar terms. For additional nursing and health care–related

Library of Congress Cataloging-in-Publication Data

Hebda, Toni.
  Internet resource guide for nurses and health care professionals /
Toni Hebda, Patricia Czar, Cynthia Mascara.– 3rd ed.
      p. ; cm.
  Includes index.
  Mascara's name appears first on the earlier ed.
  ISBN 0-13-151255-2 (alk. paper)
  1. Nursing–Computer network resources. 2. Internet. 3. Nursing informatics.
  [DNLM: 1. Internet–Resource Guides. 2. Nursing–Resource Guides.
3. Education, Distance—Resource Guides. 4. Medical Informatics–Resource Guides. 5.
Nursing Research—Resource Guides. WY 49 H443i 2005] I. Czar, Patricia. II. Mascara, Cyn-
thia. III. Title.
  RT50.5.M37 2005
  025.06'61073–dc22   2004017031

Publisher: Julie Levin Alexander
Assistant to the Publisher: Regina Bruno
Editor-in-Chief: Maura Connor
Assistant Editor: Sladjana Repic
Associate Editor: Danielle Doller
Media Editor: John J. Jordan
**Director of Production &
Manufacturing:** Bruce Johnson
Managing Production Editor: Patrick
Walsh
Production Liaison: Lakshmi
Balasubramanian
Production Editor: Heather Willison,
Carlisle Publishers Services
Manufacturing Manager: Ilene Sanford
Manufacturing Buyer: Pat Brown
Design Director: Cheryl Asherman

Design Coordinator: Maria Gugliemo-
Walsh
Cover Designer: Mary Siener
Director of Marketing: Karen Allman
Marketing Manager: Nicole Benson
Channel Marketing Manager: Rachele
Strobe
Marketing Coordinator: Janet Ryerson
Manager of Media Production: Amy
Peltier
New Media Project Manager: Tina
Rudowski
New Media Production: TSI Graphics
Composition: Carlisle Publishers Services
Cover Printer: Phoenix Color
Printing/Binder: RR Donnelley & Sons

Pearson Education Ltd.
Pearson Education Singapore, Pte. Ltd.
Pearson Education Canada, Ltd.
Pearson Education—Japan

Pearson Education Australia Pty., Limited
Pearson Education North Asia Ltd.
Pearson Educacíon de Mexico, S.A. de C.V.
Pearson Education Malaysia, Pte. Ltd.

10 9 8 7 6 5 4 3 2 1
ISBN: 0-13-151255-2

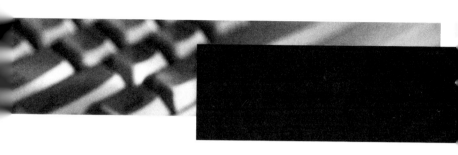

Contents

Web site addresses (URLs) and activities related to informatics and the Internet, please go to our Companion Web site at www.prenhall.com/hebda.

Toni Hebda
Patricia Czar
Cynthia Mascara

1

Introduction to the Internet for Health Care Professionals

THE INTERNET AND THE WORLD WIDE WEB

The **Internet** is a worldwide network that connects millions of computers so that they can communicate with each other. The term *Internet* was first used in the early 1980s to describe this network; today many call it simply "the Net." The exact size of the rapidly growing Internet is difficult to estimate, but its users number well into the millions. This technology first appeared in 1969 as part of a Department of Defense project to encourage researchers at different academic sites across several states to share their findings. The popularity of the Internet has increased dramatically in recent years, and the Internet now links government, universities, and commercial institutions, as well as individual users. It is neither owned nor controlled by a single agency. As a result, there is little control over the source, type, and quality of information available.

The **World Wide Web (Web or WWW)** is an information service that provides access to content on the Internet, and locates resources by address or content rather than by file names. The Web uses a system of Internet servers that support documents formatted in a special markup language called Hypertext Markup Language (HTML). HTML supports links to text, images, and sound, as well as links to other documents. Its graphical user interface (GUI) makes it simple to learn and use. You may search either by specific words or by moving from one link to another. Links are displayed by highlighted keywords, text, or images. To select a link you simply click it with your mouse button, touchpad, or trackball. The Web was first developed at the European Center for Particle Physics in Geneva as a means for scientists to publish documents while linked via the Internet. Chapter 2 discusses the functionality of the World Wide Web in more detail. The Internet and the Web expand the range of available health care information through various resources, much of which is no longer published on paper and is available only in electronic format. Some examples include research reports, practice guidelines, educational materials, and conference proceedings.

THE VALUE OF THE INTERNET

The Internet offers health care professionals and consumers the potential to increase their access to information. Much of this information is free although subscriptions may be required in some cases. Federal agencies, health care institutions, physicians, nurses, psychologists, dentists, allied health professionals, online professional journals, drug companies, equipment manufacturers, educational facilities, and discussion and chat groups offer information and advice. Users may post inquiries, read documents of commonly asked questions and answers, or search by keyword or subject. The Internet also supports online hospital services, such as registration, consumer education, appointment scheduling, telehealth, continuing education, and communication among professionals. It has even been proposed as the mechanism to support the electronic health record through a network that links health care providers, payers, and clients.

Internet services meet many of the information and communication needs of health care professionals and consumers. Although each group may use similar services and access the same sites, each has distinct goals and expectations related to using the Net.

Benefits for Health Care Professionals

The Internet encourages timely sharing of information among professionals, organizations, and alliances, as well as vendors, federal agencies, schools, and students. It decreases geographic isolation and allows professionals in remote areas to keep informed of the latest discoveries, treatment modalities, regulations, trends, and medications (including adverse reactions or interactions). Health care professionals benefit from communication with experts, listservs, and discussion and chat groups; online literature searches; and access to Web sites. These resources offer tutorials, multimedia instruction, online journals, continuing education credits, and even degree programs.

Electronic communication disseminates information quickly, allowing health care professionals to learn about revisions in practice guidelines and new study findings as soon as they are issued. The Internet provides teleconferencing capability for distance learning and continuing education. Electronic communication facilitates networking, saves time and labor through the sharing of useful tips and policies, and facilitates collaborative research and writing. The Internet even provides a forum for global mentoring, a process through which mentors in one location can facilitate the professional and personal growth of individuals in another geographic location.

Benefits for Consumers

Health care professionals need to be aware of the wealth of consumer health care information available on the Internet, as well as its growing popularity for finding this type of information. The rapid development and distribution of new knowledge means that today consumers often learn about discoveries and treatments before the professionals do because consumers are able to access many of the same sources as their health care providers. Online resources may aid in diagnosis, present new treatment options, and help consumers locate support groups.

As more people access the Internet and Web, the volume of consumer education materials and the popularity of online support groups will continue to grow. The Internet and Web offer ways to reach large numbers of people easily and inexpensively because printing costs are saved and materials can be updated quickly as needed. These features also laid the groundwork for the electronic book or **ebook**. The ebook is a file that can be downloaded to a PDA, PC, or device dedicated to the receipt and display of electronic books. Ebooks may be available at no cost but many reference books are available on file for download for a fee which includes purchase of the manuscript as well as any updates or revisions that may occur within a prescribed period of time. The American Cancer Society provides a good example of a Web site that furnishes consumer education materials. Figure 1–1 depicts a Web page found at the ACS site.

Despite their value, online resources cannot be considered a replacement for actual health care, and caution must be exercised because the data provided may not always be correct or current. Most health care providers' Web sites guide users to follow-up care. Questions about professional liability for information found on the Internet are unresolved at this time.

ACCESSING THE INTERNET

Obtaining access to the Internet may seem complex, but it need not be. The most common method of Internet access continues to be through a personal or notebook computer with a connection to the Internet through a network, such as a corporate, hospital, or university information system, or directly from a stand-alone device. Individual computers can connect to the Internet via modem using a telephone line, cable, or satellite and an Internet service provider. Wireless connectivity is also an extremely popular means to access the Internet for both notebook computers and personal digital assistants (PDAs). PDAs are specialized handheld computers that were initially used primarily to keep appointments, calendars, addresses, and telephone numbers. Advances in PDA processing capability, memory, and

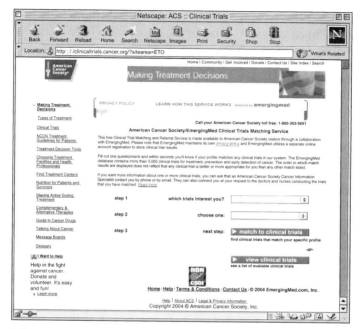

FIGURE 1–1 • American Cancer Society/EmergingMed Clinical Trials Matching Service (Reproduced with the permission of the American Cancer Society, Inc., from the ACS Web site, *http://clinicaltrials.cancer.org/?sitearea=ETO)*

design now allow these devices to send and receive e-mail and reference materials, and house common computer applications such as word processing and power point presentations. These features also make PDA use attractive as a means to access data housed on networks such as hospital information systems as well as to collect data for research and billing purposes.

Modem

A **modem** is a piece of equipment that changes computer data into pulses or signals that can be transmitted over telephone lines, cable, or satellite. It can be an external box that sits next to the computer or an internal card located within the device. Modems come in different speeds. The speed of a modem determines how quickly you can download or access information from the Internet. Because modem technology is continually improving, and speeds are getting faster, it is important to check with your local computer hardware store to see what modems are available and which one might be right for you.

Telephone Line

An ordinary telephone line can be connected to the modem. In fact, it is a simple matter to unhook a telephone from a telephone line and to connect that line to the modem. Although this method is easy and inexpensive, it is slow and callers will hear a busy signal when you are online. Solutions for those who wish to access the Internet frequently include obtaining a separate **dedicated telephone line** for use only with the modem or using a special device that splits the line, allowing incoming calls while the user is online.

Most modems are still designed to function using standard telephone lines. These phone lines are known as **analog lines**, and they transmit information using wave signals. **Digital** telephone lines, which transmit information via pulse signals, are a newer type of line that is becoming more common in business settings. If a digital line is the only type of telephone line available, you can still use your modem if you obtain a digital-to-analog jack converter box or a digital telephone with an analog modem jack. Special types of modems are required for high-speed Internet service.

Internet Service Provider

To access the Internet, you must go through an **Internet service provider** (**ISP**), which is a company that runs the computers, or servers, and software that enable you to access the Internet. In order to connect to the Internet, your modem dials the telephone number of your ISP, which then connects you to its server.

Some well-known examples of ISPs include America Online (AOL) and Microsoft Network (MSN). Many companies in the communication industry offer Internet access, including MCI and other phone companies, both local and national. Other local ISPs also exist. ISPs provide their customers with any needed software and assign each customer a unique account for Internet and World Wide Web access. When choosing an ISP, you should consider the following:

- *Price per hour.* Some ISPs allow unlimited use for a flat fee, some offer a certain amount of time per month before they begin charging extra, and some charge by the amount of time that you are online.

- *Traffic.* Find the "dial up" number (the number your modem calls to link up) of an ISP and call it at different times during the day. Some ISPs, particularly the larger companies, get a lot of traffic, and it can be difficult to get online.

- *Local telephone number.* Look for an ISP that has a local telephone number or a toll-free number for gaining Internet access (otherwise you may face a large telephone bill after using the Internet, even for only a few hours). Although large companies provide local phone numbers for many urban areas, people in rural areas may have more success finding a local telephone access number from a small local ISP. If your job requires traveling, ISPs that offer hundreds of local access numbers nationwide (e.g., AOL, MSN, and Earthlink) may better serve your needs.

- *Services provided.* Check which services the provider offers to ensure a match with your needs.

- *Support.* Determine the amount and type of technical support offered by the ISP. Some offer 24-hour support, where as others have technicians available during limited hours. Support may be provided in a variety of forms for example, by telephone, Web site, or e-mail.

- *Reliability*: Talk with other users to determine their satisfaction with their ISPs. Ask them if they ever experience problems connecting, sending and receiving e-mail, or with poor service.

High-Speed Internet Connections

Although the use of regular telephone lines for Internet access is still common for home use, other types of connections are available that offer greater speed. Local telephone companies or ISPs may provide these. **Integrated services digital network (ISDN)** lines, one of the first high-speed options, are about twice as fast as most regular phone line connections. You must contact your local phone company to have this type of line installed in your home or business, assuming it is available in your area. A special modem and other hardware is also needed. This method of Internet access is generally expensive—you will have the initial costs to install the line and to purchase the needed equipment, and then you must pay additional monthly ISDN charges to your phone company.

Another method for obtaining high-speed connections involves a **digital subscriber line (DSL)**. It has the advantage of not sharing bandwidth, thereby avoiding the decrease in transmission speeds that may occur with cable. Like ISDN and cable access, you will need special equipment, special lines, and an ISP. Your local phone company can provide information about DSL access and will charge you monthly for this access. DSL service is not available in all areas.

Cable modems have become a popular alternative for high-speed Internet connections. These special modems use the same coaxial cable that cable television signals use. This cable connects to a cable modem box, which is connected to an ethernet card in the PC. You must use a cable service provider as your ISP. This technology has the potential for high-speed connections at relatively low prices. However, a decrease in speed is a potential problem as more people in a neighborhood begin to use cable modems. This happens when the bandwidth is shared by more and more users. Still, cable modems offer an alternative means to obtaining high-speed Internet access.

Wi-fi, also known as wireless broadband, provides another means of acheiving connectivity to the Internet. Wi-fi stands for *wi*reless *fi*delity. It is wi-fi that provides "hot spots" in parks, coffee shops, fast-food restaurants, hotels, and airport lounges that allow people easily to check e-mail, instant message, or explore the World Wide Web while away from their home or office. Wi-fi uses radio signals to replace cable. Suppliers of wi-fi services hope to charge for the convenience of their service, although there is some discussion as to whether this type of connection should be free as a means to eliminate the "digital divide" between the connected Internet savvy and the less affluent, less computer literate population. The range for wi-fi is limited to approximately 150 feet. This range makes it useful for offices and older facilities where cabling costs would be prohibitive. Another new high-speed wireless data protocol, wi-max, may surplant wi-fi. Wi-max is officially known as IEEE 802.16. Critics of the wi-fi protocol express concerns for the security of its users because it is easy to spy on nearby computers. Newer security standards should help alleviate this issue. Transmitted data should be encrypted using wired equivalent privacy (WEP) or a newer encryption system called wi-fi protected access (WPA) to protect it from prying eyes. The use of virtual private networks provides another means of securing information. Connectivity is acheived because most newer computers and hand-helds include built-in wi-fi network adapters, so it is easy to get connected. Despite the many advantages associated with wireless access, it is sometimes plagued by "dead zones." These are areas where reception and transmittal of data do not occur either because devices are beyond the allowable transmission distance or signals are blocked by environmental barriers such as steel doors.

A less common method of Internet access uses satellite technology. This method requires the installation of a satellite dish, on an exterior wall or the roof for example, which is connected by cable to a special card and modem in your personal computer (PC). In some cases the user sends requests for information via land-line telephone and receives fast downloads via satellite. In other cases broadband service is two way. Satellite Internet access is available throughout most of the world through specialized ISPs. Equipment and subscription prices are more expensive than other options for Internet connectivity but provide an effective means of Internet connection, particularly for individuals in geographically remote areas.

Interactive Television

Another method of Internet access is through interactive television. This service allows subscribers to access such features as instant messaging, e-mail, headline news, sports, and weather, as well as select television programs for view.

GOING ONLINE

Once you have the necessary equipment and connectivity, you are ready to go online. "Going online" means connecting to various computer resources, such as the Internet and World Wide Web. Once you are aware of the many types of Internet resources available, you will have unlimited opportunities to find information and interact with others. Chapter 2 reviews the types of services offered through the Internet and provides information about how to access them.

2

Internet Services and Resources

The Internet provides information useful to health care professionals and consumers. This chapter discusses the wide variety of
Internet services and resources that exist to meet the information
and communication needs of these groups.

ELECTRONIC MAIL

Electronic mail (e-mail) uses computers to transmit messages
to one or more persons in remote locations almost instantaneously. Special software or programs are required to write,
send, receive, and store e-mail messages. These programs may
be housed on the user's computer, a server, or accessed via the
Web. Web-based e-mail allows the user to access and send e-mail
from any computer with an Internet connection eliminating the
need for e-mail software on the host computer. Web-based e-mail
services may be available free of charge through services such as
Hotmail, Yahoo, or Juno. Web-based e-mail may also be obtained for a fee. Other files, such as word processing documents,
spreadsheets, graphics, and photos may be attached to text
e-mails. E-mail can be sent anywhere in the world as long as the
recipient has an Internet address. Like street addresses, Internet
addresses are specific to a location and type of institution or ISP.

One of the most frequently used Internet applications, e-mail
is commonly found in private organizations, colleges and

Box 2–1

E-Mail: Advantages and Disadvantages

Advantages

- *Eliminates Telephone Tag.* Provides the ability to leave a written message.

- *Convenient.* Can be sent or retrieved from multiple locations, including work, home, or while traveling. Can be used on a 24-hour basis.

- *Easy to Prepare and Send.* Requires less effort to prepare, address, and send than the traditional means of dictation and mailing.

- *Saves Time and Money.* Eliminates postage and paper expenses.

- *Delivery Can be Almost Instantaneous.* Eliminates the time lag associated with traditional mail.

- *Messages are Time- and Date-stamped.* Provides documentation of the actual time of the mail transaction. Can also provide a log of when the message was received, read, and answered.

- *Can be Used to Transmit Other Files.* Allows you to send attached files including documents, photos, sound files, and programs.

Disadvantages

- *Interpretation of Messages Without the Benefit of Voice Inflection.* Unlike telephone conversations, e-mail eliminates the additional information that may be communicated through verbal cues.

- *High Volume of Messages Sent and Received.* The popularity of e-mail generates large numbers of messages, including copies, forwarded messages, and junk mail or spam.

- *Contamination of E-mail Attachments.* Attached files may contain a virus or worm that could infect the recipient's computer, disrupting service and access to information.

- *Security Concerns Related to Maintaining Confidentiality.* E-mail is intercepted and forwarded easily, and may be read by unintended parties. Employers have the right to read e-mail transmitted using company resources. In addition, deleted messages may be retrieved during system backups.

universities, and government agencies. Individuals may also acquire e-mail access through an ISP. This powerful connectivity tool is often the feature that first attracts users to the Internet. E-mail encourages networking among peers, yields helpful tips and shared resources, and saves time and money that would otherwise be spent in individual problem solving. E-mail is a convenient way to contact recruiters; send résumés; and keep in touch with friends, family, professional colleagues, and faculty. Box 2–1 lists some advantages and disadvantages associated with e-mail.

Components of an E-Mail Message

Every e-mail message (often called simply "an e-mail") has several standard components, regardless of the software being used. These components include the header, body, attachments, and signature.

Header   The header provides basic information about the e-mail in the following sections.

TO:	Identifies to whom the message is addressed.
CC:	Stands for "carbon copy"; lists other recipients of the message.
BCC:	Stands for "blind carbon copy"; allows the message to be received by others without their names being displayed to other recipients.
FROM:	Identifies the sender of the message.
SUBJECT:	A brief phrase describing the subject content of the e-mail.

Body   The body contains the main contents of the message as typed by the sender.

Attachments   Most e-mail software allows the sender to attach computer files. This is a handy way to share information with people in remote locations. These files may be of almost any type, including word processing documents, spreadsheets, graphic files, photos, scanned documents, sound or music, and executable files or programs. Some ISPs limit the number and size of attachments or e-mail text.

Signature Many e-mail systems allow the sender to create a standard ending for all e-mails that are sent. This "signature" may include the sender's name, address, and other identifying information.

E-Mail Addresses The recipients of the e-mail message are listed in the TO:, CC:, and BCC: fields by their e-mail addresses, not their full names. The user may see the e-mail address or, in some cases, they may see the person's name because it is stored with their e-mail address in an address book. Internet E-mail addresses are created using a standard format that indicates the person to receive the e-mail and the location or computer where that person's e-mail account can be found. The e-mail is transmitted across telephone lines, cable, satellite, wireless, or network connections to the server, which sorts the mail and sends it to the correct user.

The first part of the address is the user name of the person who should receive the e-mail, followed by an "at" (@) symbol. The remainder of the address indicates to which server and computer system the mail should be sent. The address may have additional information, such as subdomains, which identify a department or division within an organization. These are separated by periods and are listed from general to specific. An example of an Internet e-mail address is *janedoe@aol.com.* The Internet uses standard domain suffixes at the end of the e-mail address to indicate the type of organization providing the e-mail service. Some of these are listed in Box 2–2.

Many hospitals, companies, and universities provide online directories listing employees who have e-mail. The sender can select the employees by name and their e-mail addresses will be

Box 2–2 E-Mail Organizational Domains

The last portion of an e-mail address indicates the type of organization that provides the e-mail service used by the addressee. For example, $nsmith@sfhs.edu$ indicates that a user named nsmith is located at an educational organization. Country codes are two characters. Following is a partial listing of some common organizational domains:

.com	commercial organization
.edu	educational organization
.gov	government
.mil	military
.net	networking organization
.org	nonprofit organization
.ca	Canada
.th	Thailand
.uk	United Kingdom

entered automatically into the desired header field. These directories may also list groups, so that e-mail can be distributed to a particular group of people with one selection from the directory.

Some e-mail software programs allow the user to maintain a personal directory, listing the names of frequent recipients along with their e-mail addresses. When the sender clicks on a person's name, the software program will automatically enter the appropriate e-mail address. The user may also be able to build address groups with predefined members, so that e-mails can be easily addressed to a large number of people with a single selection from the directory. The user must first create a group then select the members. Specific processes may vary from one e-mail provider to another. It may be necessary to "save" the group after it is created.

Communicating with E-Mail

The popularity of e-mail has led to the informal development of abbreviations and symbols that many users include in their e-mails. These abbreviations and symbols are usually seen in informal e-mails rather than in formal business communications. **Emoticons** are symbols that are used in e-mail to express emotions or gestures. Box 2–3 lists some common abbreviations and emoticons.

Other informal terms have evolved that describe various forms of e-mail communication. Sometimes e-mail that has been returned because of an inaccurate address is referred to as undeliverable or **bounced e-mail**. Email may also bounce when the recipient has insufficient space on their server or account to accept the message or if a network failure occurs on the recipient's end. Bounced messages contain information that will indicate why the message was returned. Additional features allow the user to designate message priority or to receive confirmation that the recipient has opened his or her mail.

Managing E-Mail

Because e-mail is quite popular, users may quickly find themselves inundated with incoming mail. Therefore, when sending an e-mail message, it is important to accurately describe the contents in the subject line so that the reader can evaluate the e-mail's urgency. Be aware that readers may delete unread e-mail that appears useless or unimportant. It is important to keep current with messages to avoid being overwhelmed by large numbers of messages.

Once mail is read, the user may choose to delete it or keep it for future reference. Many e-mail systems allow the user to create directories or folders to organize and save mail. Most e-mail packages contain features that allow you to manually place messages into folders or automatically divert incoming mail into folders through the use of rules or filters using criteria such as the sender's address or specific words in the subject heading.

Box 2–3   Common E-Mail and Instant Messaging (IM) Abbreviations and Emoticons

Abbreviations

AFAIK	As far as I know	**F2F**	Face to face	**LOL**	Laughing out loud
BAK	Back at keyboard	**FWIW**	For what it's worth	**NP**	No problem
BBLR	Be back later	**GR8**	Great	**PLS**	Please
B4N	Bye for now	**GGBB**	Gotta go bye bye	**POV**	Point of view
BFO	Blinding flash of the obvious	**GMTA**	Great minds think alike	**RUOK**	Are you OK
BRB	Be right back	**H8**	Hate	**SLAP**	Sounds like a plan
BTW	By the way	**HAND**	Have a nice day	**TIA**	Thanks in advance
CTRN	Can't talk right now	**HTH**	Hope this (or that) helps	**TMI**	Too much info
CUL8R	See you later	**IMH**	In my opinion	**WB**	Welcome back
DHTB	Don't have the bandwidth	**IMHO**	In my humble opinion	**WFM**	Works for me
FAQ	Frequently asked questions	**IOW**	In other words		
FYI	For your information	**KIT**	Keep in touch		

Emoticons

:-)	smile
:-(	frown
:-O	surprise
:-D	laugh
;-)	wink

You will need to review the features of your particular software to learn how to do this. You can use rules to block, or delete, unwanted e-mail. E-mail software also allows the user to forward the message easily to other recipients or to reply to the sender. You should not forward messages unless you know that the recipient wants or needs the information. You should provide sufficient information when replying to e-mail so that the message will be clear to the recipient. In some settings, the organization deletes mail automatically after a specified time period. Users facing this situation should consider saving important message to a permanent file.

E-mail software programs list incoming e-mail by displaying information such as the date, sender, and subject. Some software may also indicate whether the e-mail has been read using symbols, boldface type, or colors. Some programs may allow the reader to sort messages by date, sender, or subject, and to search for a particular e-mail. Another feature of some programs is the ability to track when a recipient has opened an e-mail. Most e-mail packages also contain the ability to allow you to search for messages received by sender, subject, or date.

Another very important aspect in the management of e-mail is the control of spam. **Spam** is unwanted or "junk" e-mail. It wastes time and clogs e-mail systems. It is used to spread advertisements and may be used as a vehicle to disseminate malicious computer programs. Web-based e-mail packages typically include software to block spam. Anti-virus software may also include tools to eliminate the receipt of spam.

Concerns about E-Mail

As e-mail popularity grows, so do concerns related to its use. Many of these concerns involve privacy and confidentiality issues. It is important to understand that a company, university, or agency may legally read all incoming and outgoing e-mail. E-mail that has been deleted by the user in these settings may continue to exist on backup files maintained by the organization.

Another concern is that e-mail will permit malicious programs, such as viruses, worms, and Trojan horses, to be transmitted to recipients' computer equipment or systems when they are received as attachments. These malicious programs can disrupt or destroy data and are sometimes referred to as malware. Although these programs are not usually spread through the actual e-mail text or message, they may be attached to files sent with e-mail messages. However, if you scan all attachment files with up-to-date virus detection software prior to use, the threat of viruses can be minimized.

The popularity of e-mail has also resulted in a deluge of "junk mail," usually unsolicited advertisements in the form of e-mail messages. This type of message is also known as **spam**. It comprises approximately one-half of all e-mail. It eats up network bandwidth, wastes time, and drives up ISP costs. Some ISPs provide their users with utilities that allow the users to block or reduce junk mail. Whenever possible, the best way to deal with spam is to prevent it. Avoid registering for free merchandise. Do not provide your e-mail address to unfamiliar or unknown recipients. Ignore messages that read, "to be removed from this list, click here" because they are actually used by spammers to collect e-mail addresses. Do not reply to spam messages. When subscribing to services or purchasing products online, check boxes that limit with whom companies may share your information. You may consider establishing separate e-mail accounts for different purposes. Use spam filters and do not purchase products from spammers. There have been a number of efforts to block spam, including lawsuits, state and federal legislation, industry initiatives, and proposals to establish a "do not e-mail" list. Many ISPs do not sanction spam and will ban offending parties from using their services. Unfortunately, spam generally is sent through several ISPs to hide the origin so this task is not accomplished easily. Spammers often surreptitiously take over inadequately protected computers known as servers to use them to send out their messages. They rarely comply with laws that require labelling of their messages as advertisement and often make exaggerated claims for their products. In many instances spammers are located in other countries making them immune to the laws at the recipient's location. In addition to being a nuisance, some types of spam may be used to collect personal and credit card information.

Another method of dealing with spam is challenge response or **Captcha**, software. This special software works by asking the e-mail sender to answer a question or complete a task that requires human intervention. No mail is accepted unless its validity has been confirmed by a human being. Captcha stands for completely automatic public Turing test to tell computers and humans apart. Challenge response tools are effective in filtering out spam but they create additional network traffic. Some informal rules for using e-mail efficiently and safely are listed in Box 2–4.

Instant messaging (IM) is an Internet service that allows users to carry on a conversation in "real time," much the same as any other conversation. Therefore, all participants are con-

---

Box 2–4 **Informal Rules for E-Mail Use**

- Change password for e-mail access immediately after it is first assigned and frequently thereafter.

- Limit copies to the people who need the information. This keeps the number of messages manageable.

- Choose an accurate description for the subject line. This practice helps recipients to determine which messages should be read first.

- Give e-mail messages the same consideration given to business correspondence. E-mail may be seen by parties other than the intended recipients. In an e-mail message, nothing should be written that you would not publicly post.

- Make messages clear, brief, and to the point.

- Avoid the use of all capital letters. They are difficult to read, and may be perceived as yelling, according to e-mail etiquette.

- Limit abbreviations to those that are easily understood.

- Read mail, file messages in categories, and delete messages no longer needed on a regular basis. This frees storage space and helps optimize system functioning, as well as making it easier to find and retrieve messages later.

- Use mechanisms to prevent unwanted or junk mail.

nected to the Internet at the same time, which distinguishes this service from e-mail. Messaging may be conducted privately between two people, or among a small group. A statement or response is typed by the user and is almost instantly available to other users connected to the instant messaging service. The immediacy of IM makes it extremely popular for business and personal use. It is also possible to conduct other tasks while engaging in IM. IM follows an earlier form of online chat known as **Internet Relay Chat (IRC)** that remains very popular today. Instant messaging services often provide special groups or locations, called chat rooms, for the discussion of a specific topic. You can find special interest chats by searching the Web, talking to friends, and exploring specialty portals. Nursechat.com is one site that provides opportunities for live chat. Yahoo! maintains a number of chats listing them by category. The health and wellness category is broken down into several different groups. IM has given rise to its own language. Box 2–3 lists abbreviations commonly used in e-mail and IM. You should familiarize yourself with common IM abbreviations before starting to chat.

A benefit of IM is that it provides a degree of anonymity, which allows users the freedom to ask questions or make statements that may be of a confidential nature. However, this same anonymity also allows users to deliberately portray themselves as someone else. For this reason you should leave your personal profile information blank or provide fictitious information to avoid being the target of stalkers and identity thieves. IM is also available free of charge.

Communicating with IM

IM requires a connection to the Internet, an account with one of the major IM services, and IM client software. Four major IM services are Instant Messenger (AIM) and ICQ which are both owned by America Online, Microsoft's Messenger, and Yahoo! Messenger. Each of these services offers the capability for one-on-one or multiparty text chat and file transfer. In some cases it is also possible to participate in voice chats or videoconference with similarly outfitted participants. You can determine who can and cannot send you messages, and whether you appear available to chat. You can create contact lists and only accept messages from these persons. Despite these capabilities, the major IM services do not communicate so it is not possible to chat with persons from other IM services. Most IM services use peer-to-peer technology, which means that once conversations begin there is no administrative ability to control conversations in process or archive them.

Concerns about Instant Messaging

In addition to the lack of ability to exchange messages between users of different IM programs, there are also concerns related to authenticity, the law, security, accountability, and spim. **Spim** refers to unsolicited IM, often containing a link to a Web site that the spimmer is trying to market.

Public IM systems do not validate the authenticity of users or capture transcripts of messages. This can lead to issues with the exchange of potentially sensitive information as occurs in health care where exchange of information must be limited to a need-to-know basis and must be adequately protected from inadvertent disclosure. Electronic messaging is considered to be on par with paper documents legally. This brings with it requirements for retention as well as considerations for how information that it contains may be used. Corporate use of IM requires the development of the infrastructure to support it. The peer-to-peer technology of IM currently allows participants to bypass administrative safeguards to institutional computer systems. This presents the very real danger that viruses and worms may be introduced, threatening the system and the information that it houses. There are also issues related to accountability. The majority of IM programs are the free programs already noted. Use in the office generally occurs as employees take it on themselves to download and use the software. Organizations need to establish and enforce policies on the appropriate use of IM. Companies may be held liable for messages that are found to be profane or inappropriate in nature.

LISTSERVS

A **listserv** is actually an e-mail subscription list. A mailing list program copies and distributes all e-mail messages to subscribers. All mail goes through a central computer that acts as the server for the list. Some groups have a moderator who first screens messages for relevance. Listservs, which are sometimes referred to as discussion groups, mailing lists, or electronic conferences, provide information on thousands of topics. A complete list of listservs may be obtained by sending the request "lists global" to any listserv or by searching the Tile.net Internet reference online at *http://www.tile.net*, which lists more than 90,000 listservs. A list of some specific listservs and their addresses can be found on the Companion Web site at *www.prenhall.com/hebda*.

In order to subscribe to a listserv, individuals must send the e-mail message "sub" or "subscribe," followed by their first and last names. Exact commands vary. Each listserv sends explicit instruction for subscription, posting messages, and terminating subscription to new subscribers. Most listservs provide help and instructions on request. Subscribers may participate in discussions or simply monitor them. Listserv participants should read their mail frequently and skim messages for subjects of interest to keep up with discussions. Subscribers may terminate their participation at any time by sending an "unsubscribe" e-mail message.

FILE TRANSFER

File transfer is the ability to move files from one location to another across the Internet. Although small files may be transferred as attachments to e-mail, file transfer may be used to transfer larger files. In fact, some ISPs ask their customers not to send large files via e-mail because this can impede performance. In these cases, transferring files over the Internet is preferred. Users may download archived files that they find interesting or give their files to others. Transferred files can include graphics, text, or computer programs. The actual movement of data is accomplished through the **file transfer protocol** (**FTP**). FTP is a set of instructions that controls both the physical transfer of data across the network and its appearance on the receiving end. The benefit of file transfer is that users working on a group project can view work developed by others. FTP may be available independently or as a component of some World Wide Web software. Internet etiquette calls for FTP execution after peak business hours to prevent slow response times when using computer resources in a business or educational setting. Directions for the access and use of FTP may be found under the Help tab of your Web browser. Binary file transfer (BFT) represents another standard for file transfer.

WORLD WIDE WEB

The World Wide Web (Web or WWW) is an information service that can access data by content and support a multimedia approach. The Web's graphical user interface makes it the most user friendly service on the Internet. The Web provides a forum for the exchange of ideas, free marketing, and public relations. Box 2–5 lists advantages and disadvantages associated with using the World Wide Web.

One particularly popular Web feature is the **home page**, the first page seen at a particular Web site. The home page presents general information about a topic, person, or organization. Web sites may consist of a single page or hundreds of pages of information linked together. They vary in complexity from simple text pages to pages with elaborate graphics, sound, and video. Figure 2–1 displays the Prentice Hall nursing home page.

Web pages are written in **HyperText Markup Language** (**HTML**). This language includes text as well as graphics, video, and sound files. HTML provides special instructions for how text will be displayed, and how video and sound will be accessed. It also can include highlighted references or links to

Box 2–5	Using the World Wide Web: Advantages and Disadvantages

Advantages

- Browser software is available for all types of computers.
- Easy to use.
- Supports text, pictures, video, and sound.
- The amount of information available on the Web is constantly expanding.
- Decreases Internet overload because it links to other documents instead of including them as attachments.
- Eliminates need to hold a line open while a document is read because the document can be transferred to the host computer and the connection is terminated.
- Facilitates document transfer.
- May support voice communications.

Disadvantages

- No one person or group controls the Web, just as no one controls the Internet; this results in a wide variation of quality and accuracy of material.
- Documents may not supply sufficient depth in content.
- Not all Web pages display a date of authorship, the author's credentials, or information about how to contact the author or organization.
- Web sites may change without leaving a "forwarding address."
- Vulnerable to hacker attacks.
- Employers may be concerned over wasted company time and lost productivity as people explore the Web.

other documents that the user may choose if additional information about a topic is desired.

Links, also known as hypertext, are words or phrases distinguished from the remainder of the document through the use of underlining or a different text color. In addition to text links, pictures or icons may be used in the same way. Links allow users

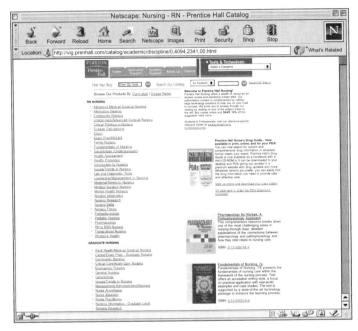

FIGURE 2–1 • Home Page of the Prentice Hall Nursing Division (Reproduced with permission, Prentice Hall Health. From the Prentice Hall Health site *http://vig.prenhall.com/catalog/academic/discipline/0,4094,2341,00.html*.)

to skip from point to point within or among documents. Clicking on links with the mouse allows the user to be seamlessly transported to another area of the document or another Web site. In many cases, the color of the link is changed after the user has clicked on it to indicate that it has been used.

World Wide Web Addresses

Every Web site has a specific address, called a **uniform resource locator** (URL). The URL indicates the name of the document, as well as its Web location and the type of server on which it resides. The first part of the URL indicates the protocol or server type that is used to retrieve the document, followed by a colon. Some protocols include HyperText Transfer Protocol (HTTP), FTP, and various news server protocols. The rest of the address indicates the domain name of the computer that contains the document. The URL is usually listed in the header of the browser software.

Information for Health Care Professionals

Health care professionals may use the World Wide Web to learn more about any of the following topics:

- *Undergraduate, graduate, and doctoral degree programs.* Many schools have Web pages that provide information about their philosophies, curricula, and application processes. In some cases potential candidates may be able to complete applications online. Increasing numbers of schools offer Web-based instruction. This may be a part of a traditional course, a stand-alone course, or an entire program.

- *Professional associations.* Many groups, including the American Nurses Association, maintain Web sites that discuss the purpose of the group and advantages of membership. This increases visibility for the group and serves as a recruitment strategy to attract new members. These sites may also include links to other sites of interest.

- *Nursing, medical, and health care informatics.* Announcements of upcoming meetings and calls for papers about informatics can be found on the Web, as well as information about the field.

- *Online journals.* Some traditional journals offer electronic versions of their publications in addition to the printed version; other journals are offered only in an electronic format.

- *Continuing education offerings.* Program announcements and even entire courses may be found on the Web.

- *Disease-specific information and recommended treatment modalities.* A number of special interest or disease-focused agencies maintain Web sites.
- *Employment opportunities.* Health care professionals may use the Web to conduct job searches, create and distribute résumés, complete online job applications, and research information about potential employers.

The Companion Web site at *www.prenhall.com/hebda* provides a list of nursing Web sites, as well as related sites of interest.

Information for Consumers

Some practitioners provide information on the Web as a public service. MD Advice.com maintains an "Ask an Expert" section where you can pose a question or review an archive of previous questions and answers. Web4Health offers Free Online Medical Advice Answers providing more than 700 questions about psychology, mental health, and relationships by a team of experts. There are also sites that provide advice for a fee. Professional organizations also provide health information for the public. The American Medical Association Web site offers a section for patients with links to health information, answers about medical services in their community, publications, and lists of practitioners in their area. Most nonprofit organizations also provide health information. The American Heart Association, the American Cancer Society, and the National Cancer Institute are among the growing list of groups that maintain Web sites. There are also a large number of government sites that provide credible health information. These include the National Library of Medicine, Medicare, the Veteran's Administration, Healthfinder, FirstGov for Seniors, the U.S. Food and Drug Administration, the Federal Trade Commission, and the United States Department of Agriculture, to name a few. Many hospitals and health-care networks, pharmaceutical companies, and drug store chains also provide information on common health conditions and diagnostic tests as a public relations tool. The volume of available health information is staggering. Consumers need to exercise caution in evaluating the credibility and currency of information found on the Web.

BROWSERS

A **browser** is software that accesses the World Wide Web and allows the user to move easily from site to site. Browsers may be obtained from an ISP or a computer store, or may come bundled with other software loaded on the PC at the time of sale. Web use increased after the introduction of Mosaic, the first browser. Netscape Navigator, Microsoft's Internet Explorer, and AOL are the predominant browers at this time. RapidBrowser XP, Mozilla, and Opera provide alternatives. Browsers commonly distribute ads but ad-free versions are available for a fee.

There are still many things that browsers do not do. Additional programs are constantly being developed to fill this void. These applications are designed to view graphics or video, construct Web pages, play sounds, or even remotely control another PC over the Internet. These programs are often available on the Web at no cost and are often written in Java. Java is a programming language that enables the display of moving text, animation, and musical excerpts on Web pages.

SEARCH TOOLS

Several search tools, such as **search indexes, search engines,** and **meta search tools** available to help users find information on the Web. With these programs the user can search the Web for pages or documents by topic without knowing specific URLs. These powerful tools provide the user with many search options. Each tool maintains its own index or list of information on the Web and uses its own method of organizing topics. Because of this variation in organization, searches conducted with different tools yield different results. The distinction between the different types of tools is blurry. In general search indexes are appropriate when general information is requested. Search indexes, otherwise known as subject guides or directories, organize Web sites by topic. Yahoo! is an example of a general search index. Search indexes are appropriate when you are looking for broad information. Two examples or health-related sites that provide subject guides include HealthWeb and Allnurses.com. Search engines use automated programs that search the Web, compiling a list of links to sites relevant to keywords supplied by the user. The search may also include a type of discussion forum conducted on the Web known as news groups or usenet discussions. Search engines are indicated when it is necessary to find a specific topic. Google and AltaVista are examples of search engines. Although subtle differences exist among each, all permit the user to enter a search word or phrase. For example, information about a disease may be located by symptom, disease name, drug interaction, or support-related groups.

After the user enters the topic, Web sites that contain the search item are displayed. The number of "hits," or Web sites that carry this word or phrase, varies according to the search tool used. Enclosing key phrases in quotation marks or parentheses may improve search results; otherwise, all documents containing portions of the key phrase will be identified. Search help pages are available to aid users with their search strategies. Until recently, retrieval of comprehensive results meant repeating a search several times with different search engines to identify all relevant sites. Now **metasearch tools** shorten search time by employing several engines at once, yielding more comprehensive data in less time. Examples of search tools and unifiers are listed in Box 2–6.

Search Strategies

The use of search tools to find specific information on the Web can be both effective and frustrating. Search tools weight pages so that the most commonly useful links are displayed first. There are several ways to weight pages, but the best-known

Box 2–6
Examples of Internet Search Tools

Search Engine	URL
AltaVista	*http://www.altavista.com*
ClusterMed	*http://vivisimo.com/clustermed*
Excite	*http://www.excite.com*
Google	*http://www.google.com*
HotBot	*http://www.hotbot.lycos.com*
Lycos	*http://www.lycos.com*
Medical World Search	*http://www.mwsearch.com*
Open Directory Project	*http://www.dmoz.org*
Yahoo!	*http://www.yahoo.com*

Metasearch Engines

AskJeeves	*http://www.ask.com*
Copernic	*http://www.copernic.com*
Dogpile	*http://www.dogpile.com*
Highway61	*http://www.highway61.com*
Ixquick	*http://ixquick.com*
Mamma	*http://www.mamma.com*
Metacrawler	*http://www.metacrawler.com*
NewsTrawler	*http://www.newstrawler.com/nt/nt_home.html*
ProFusion	*http://www.profusion.com*
Search	*http://www.search.com*
Teoma	*http://www.directhit.com/*
The BigHub	*http://www.TheBigHub.com*
Vivisimo	*http://vivisimo.com*
WebCrawler	*http://www.webcrawler.com*

method is based on the popularity of each site as represented by the number of other sites that link to it. Enclosing key phrases in quotation marks is recommended as a way to obtain better results with some, but not all, search tools, otherwise all documents containing portions of the key phrase will be identified. The relevance of search results is also determined by whether the search engine is ad sponsored. Many results contain links that advertisers have paid the search engine to display prominently. Paid links are labeled as advertisements by some tools, whereas others include them among overall search results. Because of this practice, you may find that search results obtained with certain tools may not meet your purposes. Many metasearch tools fail to label paid links. Portal sites may also rank their affiliated products and services highly in search results. Consumer groups have asked the Federal Trade Commission (FTC) to look at this issue. Try several tools to see which ones best serve your purposes. Librarians can also provide information on specialized search tools. Federated, or cross-database, search tools can search library catalogs, commercial abstracting and indexing databases, Web search engines, and a variety of other databases.

Because of the immense amount of information available, a broad search may yield so many hits that you cannot sift through them to find relevant information. The following search strategies will greatly increase the success of your searches and, therefore, the usefulness of the Internet as a resource for you:

- *Use keywords.* Using several words or a phrase optimizes your chance of finding what you are looking for.
- *Use connectors.* Use "and" to find information related to two keywords. Use "not" to exclude information about a keyword.
- *Use plus and minus signs.* Placing a plus sign (+) before a keyword indicates that this word must be included in the results. Preceding a keyword with a minus sign (−) indicates that it should not be included.

- *Use the Bookmark feature.* This button (or its equivalent, such as Favorite Places for AOL users) creates shortcuts to a favorite site that can be easily accessed for future visits.

- *Use the Back button to retrace your steps.* This button will bring you back to previous Web pages visited during the current session.

- *Use the History feature.* This shows a list of Web pages that you have visited previously in the current session and allows you to go back to one quickly without having to retrace your steps.

- *Use the Help function associated with your search engine.* Specific features described in the Help function may aid you in efficiently using the search engine.

- *Turn off graphics.* This will help to speed up searches.

- *Use the first few results listed.* If your search yields many sources, the first 10 are usually the most relevant.

- *Use a search unifier.* This is more effective than using a single search engine.

- *Use advanced search features.* These features allow you to limit the search by date, language, file format, type of site, and/or exact phrase for more specific results.

You may still miss information when you conduct a search because results are not available in the language searched, information is password protected or stored in formats that are not indexed, or because content incorporates multiple concepts making it difficult to index. It is still necessary to search databases to locate detailed literature and research reports on specific areas. While it is possible to access many databases from home, many require access codes and fees unless they are accessed through your local academic or community library.

NEWS GROUPS

Another popular Internet feature is **usenet news groups**. These discussion groups are similar to listservs in content and diversity.

More than 100,000 discussion groups exist, each dedicated to a different topic. These groups provide a forum where any user can post e-mails for discussion and reply. Users do not pay to subscribe to these groups, and they do not receive individual e-mails. Instead, they may participate at any time free of charge. (ISPs) do not carry every news group. ISP administrators decide which news groups will be available to their customers and how long messages will be stored. Only e-mails that are currently stored on the user's ISP computer may be read. Older messages are automatically deleted. Special programs called **news reader software** are needed by the individual users to read messages posted on the news group. Many different news readers are available, and they usually come bundled with Web browsers. It is also possible to subscribe to services such as Supernews (*http://www.supernews.com*) for full access to usenet groups. This type of service promises fast access, complete access to all usenet groups, and longer retention of messages for reader convenience for a nominal fee. Some examples of nursing usenet groups include the following:

- *Sci.med.nursing.* This is a general forum for the discussion of all types of nursing issues. A review of discussion topics reveals current concerns in the profession by country and practice area. Individual nurses may request assistance with particular problems and receive help from people across the globe.

- *Alt.npractitioners.* Issues pertaining to nurse practitioners provide the focus for this group.

- *Bit.listserv.snurse-l.* This is a group for international nursing students.

The first part of a news group name indicates the hierarchy, or category, of topics. The major hierarchies include the following:

- *Alt.* Stands for "alternative" and indicates topics that are not official.

- *Biz.* Topics deal with business products, services, or reviews.
- *Comp.* Topics include computer-related issues.
- *Humanities.* Topics include fine art, literature, and philosophy.
- *Misc.* Stands for "miscellaneous" and includes health, fitness, employment, and classified notices.
- *News.* Topics concern the news groups.
- *Rec.* Topics concern recreation, sports, games, collecting, music, and art.
- *Sci.* Scientific topics include chemistry, biology, and medicine.
- *Soc.* Social issues include politics, religion, and human rights.
- *Talk.* Topics include debates about an issue.

No single person is in charge of universal usenet procedures, but informal rules and etiquette for participants have developed. The first rule is that all new users should read the **frequently asked questions** (**FAQ**) document before sending any messages of their own. The FAQ file serves to introduce the group, update new users on recent discussions, and eliminate repetition of questions. Additional usenet guidelines call for the following:

- *Short postings.* This helps to maintain interest while preventing any individual or subgroup from monopolizing the group.
- *No sensationalism.* The intent of usenet groups is the sharing of information, not gossip.
- *No outright sales.* Usenet originated in academia and relies on a cooperative environment. Advertising, by custom, is kept at a minimum.
- *Respect for the group focus.* Posting messages that are not relevant wastes time and resources.

News groups may be discovered through any of the following methods: searching the Web by topic, word of mouth from individuals with common interests, conferences, professional publications, or searching through lists of all available news groups. If no news group exists for a given topic, instructions on how to start one can be found on the Internet.

BLOGS

A **blog** is a frequent chronological publication of personal thoughts and Web links, as defined at *http://www.marketingterms. com/dictionary/blog*. Other terms for blogs include "Web logs" or "Weblogs." Many people think of a blog as an online journal that describes what is happening in a person's life as well as what is happening on the Web. A number of automated blog publishing sites are now available to assist the blogger. One of the most well known sites is Blogger at *blogger.com*. Blog is an abbreviation for Web log.

Content varies widely from personal diaries, to requests for contributions and special interest blogs organized by topics. Blogs provide an informal way to talk with other persons sharing common interests. Blogs have spread to the business world as a means to talk to customers, employees, and vendors providing marketing opportunities. The disadvantage of this approach is that it can also create a tone that puts off readers. Blogs are supposed to be spontaneous. This can create problems when they are used as forums for institutions because posted material may contain questionable material or comments that may be perceived as offensive. Blogs have been incorporated into courses at some schools as a means to facilitate learning. Blogs provide a means for students to build an online classrroom community, provide feedback to faculty, extend class discussions and aid collaboration with peers.

BULLETIN BOARD SYSTEMS

Bulletin board systems (BBSs) allow users to make announcements, share files, and post questions. Originally, BBSs differed from listserv and usenet groups because Internet access was not required. Instead participants dialed in directly via a modem connection. Web sites have largely replaced this form of BBS. A moderator determines what e-mails will be placed on the BBS. One example of this updated type of bulletin board is the All-nurses.com bulletin board at *http://allnurses.com/forums/index*.

3

Common Concerns Related to Internet Use

Now that you know what the Internet is and some of the services that it offers, we'll examine basic user rules, known as "netiquette" as well as common concerns that surround its use.

NETIQUETTE

Netiquette is just like it sounds: etiquette on the Internet. It is simply basic, common courtesy to others. Because no single person owns or controls the Internet, individual users must be facilitative and kind when participating in discussion groups, authoring Web pages, or sending e-mail, instant or text messages. The following list contains general netiquette standards for online communication.

- *Do not make assumptions.* Avoid one-word responses. Do not assume that the recipient remembers the original question or statement to which you are responding. Avoid abbreviations that are not commonly known.

- *Do not be judgmental.* Be professional and careful in what you write. E-mail is easily forwarded to others and can be printed. Instant messages may be shown to other people. Word statements carefully to prevent misinterpretation.

Flaming is the use of angry and insulting language directed at a particular person or group.

- *Proofread your messages carefully.* Poor grammar and spelling reflect badly on the sender.

- *Be timely in your replies.* This is simple courtesy.

- *Use attachments wisely.* Check with recipients before sending an attachment to determine whether they have the needed software to access it. Large files may take a long time to download, and the recipient may prefer to receive this information in another format. One alternative is to "zip" or compress large files before attaching them. Special software is needed to do this and to open files for the recipient.

- *Make postings brief and to the point.* Recipients may not read lengthy e-mail messages or postings.

- *Use online communication appropriately.* Do not send chain letters or mass distribution letters unless you know that recipients want to receive them. Mass mailing of unsolicited "junk" mail (*spamming*) can be quite annoying for recipients. Exercise judgement when forwarding mail. Not everyone feels a "need-to-know."

- *Do not use all capital letters.* This practice, known as shouting or screaming, is difficult to read and is considered rude.

- *Respect others.* Read the frequently asked questions (FAQ) before participating in listserv or other group discussions to avoid unnecessary repetition. Be forgiving of other people's mistakes.

CONCERNS RELATED TO INTERNET USE

There are a number of concerns related to the use of the Internet. The biggest issues are information security and quality; lost time and productivity related to computer viruses and worms, spam; and spim; information overload and identity theft. Another major concern in health care is HIPPA compliance. A lesser, but still important, matter is learning what is considered proper conduct when navigating in cyberspace. **Cyberspace** is the term used to refer to the online world created by computer systems.

Internet Security

Security concerns surrounding the use of the Internet and World Wide Web include (1) the fear that outside persons or agencies may gain access to information that should be secure, (2) the fear that computer systems may suffer damage either from computer viruses or from hackers, and (3) identity theft.

Unauthorized access to information is a concern for all individuals and agencies. Many people are afraid that the use of computers, particularly with Internet access, allows others to see, and possibly seize, information on their computers. The open nature of the Internet makes private computer networks with Internet access vulnerable to this threat. For this reason, private computer networks generally use a combination of hardware and software known as a *gateway* to connect to larger networks. A **gateway** provides a means to screen Internet messages before they are permitted to enter the private network.

A **firewall** is one type of gateway designed to protect private network resources from outside hackers, network damage, and theft or misuse of information. Users should not be aware of the presence of a firewall. Although they are designed to protect you, firewalls may be a source of frustration if they prevent access to certain Web sites. If this is a problem, talk to the technical support staff in your organization or review the settings for your own software. At one time individual PC users did not need to worry about this level of protection unless they transmitted sensitive data or left their computers connected to other computer systems for lengthy periods. The frequency of port attacks and rise in the incidence of cybercrime make firewall protection important for everyone using the Internet. Firewall software may be available through antivirus software vendors. Port attacks occur when hackers looking for unprotected computer connections to the Internet attempt to access that connection to view and use information contained on that computer or its network. In some cases hackers may take over the computer for their own use. An example of this is seen when the captured computer is used to house pornographic Web sites or send unsolicited e-mail without the user's knowledge. **Cybercrime** commonly refers to the use of computers to steal stored personal information, such as social security numbers, credit card numbers, and bank PIN. Health care providers and institutions need precautions to protect medical record data.

Another strategy for protecting sensitive information is **encryption.** This process uses special software to encode the information or data before it is transmitted across the Internet, which provides a safeguard from unauthorized view. Authorized recipients have software that reverses the coding process, allowing the information to be accessed.

Another concern for people using the Internet is that they will get a computer virus, worm, or Trojan horse infection when Internet and World Wide Web resources are accessed. A **virus** is a malicious program that can disrupt or destroy data, with effects that range from annoying to destructive. Relatively benign viruses may flash a message across the screen as the user works whereas destructive viruses destroy information and shut down entire computer systems. A **worm** is a virus that replicates, or makes copies of, itself. It may be passed to other computers in the form of a joke program or some other software program. A **Trojan horse** is a destructive program that masquerades as a benign application. Unlike viruses, Trojan horses do not replicate themselves, but they can be just as damaging. One of the most insidious types of Trojan horse is a program that claims to rid your computer of viruses but instead introduces viruses onto your computer.

Computer viruses may be contracted from the Internet and World Wide Web when files are downloaded and opened for use.

For example, it is quite common to send files as attachments to e-mail messages. Good computing practices lessen the risk of contracting a virus. One should not open file attachments if their origins are unknown. The next best way to deal with file attachments is to scan them for viruses prior to opening them. Files that are downloaded from the Web should also be scanned with the most recent **antivirus software** prior to use. It is also possible to contract harmful software, or malware, when visiting a Web site that contains hidden, malicious code. This is known as a browser attack, browser-based attack, or browser hi-jacking. This type of attack can be avoided by not clicking on Web sites listed in spam and by changing browser settings. Internet Explorer (IE) has been vulnerable to this type of attack for the following reasons. First it is the predominant browser used by the majority of the public. Secondly, its' default settings allow the launching of ActiveX controls. ActiveX is a set of technologies developed by Microsoft. IE security settings can be changed by choosing the following menu items: Tools, Internet Options, the Security tab, and finally the security level. The security level should be set to medium or higher. This setting prompts the user to authorize the downloading of potentially unsafe content. This will prevent the hidden launch of ActiveX controls. You need to know that changing your security settings may alter the way that desired Web sites respond as well. Competing browsers have not been subject to as many attacks primarily because they support the Java and JavaScript programming languages instead of ActiveX. You may protect yourself from a browser attack by disabling JavaScript. The method to accomplish this varies slightly by browser but look for a "preferences" option then uncheck the box that indicates Java is enabled. There are browser checkup sites that you may visit to learn about new threats. Scanit's Browser Security Test *(http://www.scanit.be/en/index.htm.)* and Qualys' Free Browser Checkup *(http://browsercheck.qualys.com/)* are two examples of such sites. For more information about computer security and viruses, visit the Computer Security Resource Center

(CSRC) at *http://csrc.nist.gov/virus*, the CERT Coordination Center *(http://www.cert.org/other_sources/viruses.html)*, or the home pages maintained by antivirus software companies such as Symantec or Mcafee.

Privacy Concerns

There is a growing concern among Internet users that their privacy is violated by software that tracks the Web sites that they have visited and accesses information that they have provided, which can be used to obtain sensitive information contained on their computers. The simplest type of tracking software creates a "cookie" on your computer when you visit certain Web sites. A **cookie** is a text file that is saved on your computer in a folder in your browser's directory and is available in active memory while your browser is running. A cookie may store information about the sites that you have visited, and may be used to personalize the information that is available on some Web sites or to track user demographics. Cookies are not dangerous to your computer; they are simple text files that can be read using a text editor program or word processor. Cookies can make it easier for you to access online updates to your antivirus software as well as expedite entry to regularly visited Web sites.

Cookies present a threat to your privacy only if you provide personal information to a Web site, and that site stores it in the form of a cookie. More information about cookies can be found at the Cookie Central Web site at *www.cookiecentral.com*. When visiting Web sites it is wise to read any disclosure statements that may address how your private information is handled. You should also be careful about the type of information that you provide and provide personal or sensitive information only to those sites that ensure encryption and have dependable reputations. You can control the creation of cookies by changing the privacy setting on your browser. This may be found in the Tools menu under Internet options.

Another type of tracking software is known as spyware. **Spyware** tracks surfing habits and may bombard you with ads or even load software that sends information stored on your computer to other parties. It may have come piggybacked on downloaded Internet software. Spyware is sometimes also referred to as adware, sneakware or snoopware. Spyware threatens information security, devours network resources, crashes PCs, and generates more spam by sending e-mail addresses that it finds back over the Internet to be traded, shared, or sold to spammers. Antispyware software is now available. You can also minimize your exposure to spyware by keeping Windows, Internet Explorer, and antivirus software up-to-date; using discretion when downloading software; installing a firewall; changing settings to prevent entry of executable e-mail attachments; and not clicking on Web links found in spam.

Yet another threat to privacy is identity (ID) theft. One of the fastest-growing scams on the Internet is the use of "urgent e-mail" that asks you to divulge personal information such as social security numbers, passwords for online accounts, and credit card information. Most look legitimate and may even include links to Web sites that look like bank, credit card, or merchant Web sites. This particular approach is sometimes called "**phishing**." It is easy to perpetrate and presents a low risk of getting caught. Do not respond to suspicious e-mail and do not click on any Web links contained in suspicious e-mail. Instead forward phishing e-mail to the FTC site at *UCEFTC.gov*. If you have responded to phishing e-mail, immediately contact your banks or credit card companies to try to prevent the misuse of account information. Obtain a copy of your credit report to help ensure that nothing unusual is happening. You may also file an ID theft complaint at the FTC's site, *www.consumer.gov/idtheft*. If you believe that personal information is being misused, ask that a fraud alert be placed on your credit files so that no creditor can authorize new credit without first contacting you. Visit *www.antiphishing.org* for tips to avoid becoming a victim.

Evaluating Online Information

The Internet offers a wealth of information, but not all of it is valid, current, or without bias. The very nature of the Internet allows information to be posted quickly and often without the review or approval of any controlling bodies. This removes the normal safeguards found with materials that undergo the editorial review imposed by publishers. At present there is no consistent system for evaluation or review of Web information although several groups are looking at the quality of posted materials, including most professional organizations, the Health Internet Ethics (Hi-Ethics) Alliance, the Health on the Net Foundation (HON), HealthWeb, Healthfinder, the Healthcare Coalition, the American Accreditation Health Care Commission (URAC), the European Council, and the World Health Organization. None of these groups impose mandatory controls over quality. Hi-Ethics published a set of 14 principles in 2000 that forms the basis for URAC accreditation. Sites that have URAC accreditation display a seal. The seal indicates that the site meets more than 50 standards, which include disclosure, site policies and structure, content currency and accuracy, linking, privacy, security, and accountability. Although URAC accreditation ensures the quality of posted material, there is an abundance of online material that has never been reviewed for accreditation. When reviewing online materials, you need to make your own decisions on the quality of information that is found.

Sophisticated search tools can locate material efficiently but they do not guarantee information quality. Health care professionals and consumers should evaluate online resources with the same criteria they apply to other sources of information. The following list suggests specific areas to look for when evaluating online information:

- *Credentials of the source.* Large professional associations, such as hospitals, universities, government, and official health organizations, tend to have the most reliable sites. In some cases the source is not readily apparent. For example, it is important to consider whether information provided mirrors the focus of professional education and expertise. You can determine whether that source has the authority to address the topic. For example, does the author have education and experience in the field? Unfortunately, not all Web sites identify a source or provide information about the background of the individual or organization.

- *The ability to validate information.* Validation of information can be difficult unless the source can be traced to a reputable university or other agency. Many messages and Web sites identify a person or persons to contact for further information. When facts and studies are cited, the original source should be stated so users can review it and draw their own conclusions. It should also be possible to corroborate information from independent sources.

- *Accuracy.* No controlling body verifies the accuracy of information that is placed on the Internet. Postings should identify the contact person or site references that can be checked to provide verification of information. The origin of information should be identified so that the reader understands whether it is opinion or fact.

- *Date of issue or revision.* One problem with the Internet and World Wide Web is that not all sites contain dates indicating when material was written, revised, or reviewed, making it difficult to determine whether information is current. Check sites for some indication of the most recent update.

- *Bias of the posting organization or person.* Commercial uses of the Internet are growing daily. The consumer must determine whether information is biased in favor of a particular product or commercial service. Advertising or product promotion may be more difficult to identify on the Internet than in traditional printed publications or television. There is also an issue of sponsorship. Although many Web sites started because someone believed that the content belonged on the Internet, ongoing maintenance generally requires that sites be self-sustaining or receive sponsorship.

- *Comprehensiveness.* It is important to determine whether enough information is available to provide an overall view on a topic. The ability to link to other Web sites and sources of information can facilitate comprehensiveness if it is used properly.

- *Comparable sources.* One means of evaluating information is to check other sites to see if they reflect similar content.

- *Intended purpose/audience.* Web pages should clearly state their purposes and intended audiences. There are, for example, sites geared toward health care consumers and other sites that are written for health care professionals. These sites vary in level of writing and use of terminology.

- *Ease of navigation.* Content should be well organized with appropriate use of hyperlinks. All links should be to current Web pages and download easily.

- *Disclaimers.* Sites that express individual opinions should contain a statement to that effect to help users distinguish between fact and opinion.

- *Site accreditation.* Several groups have been working to ensure the quality of information found on health-related Web sites. As a consequence of these efforts some sites display a "seal" such as the URAC seal, that indicates that their sites meet a set of predetermined standards for the quality of information posted. Compliance is purely voluntary.

- *Privacy policies.* Sites that collect personal information need to identify how that information may be used so that visitors can determine whether to disclose information.

Information Overload

The number of e-mails, instant and text messages, Faxes, and online information escalates daily. While many people see the unlimited access to online information as an opportunity, others find themselves affected by information overload. **Information overload** results when there is too much information produced too quickly, some of which is contradictory, to make a decision or remain informed about a topic. Information overload is a problem for persons who lack the focus and tools to determine what information is credible, current, relevant to their situation, and comes from a reliable source. Information overload can be a problem for health care consumers and professionals who try to address questions based upon information found online. It is important to help consumers and peers locate quality information and to exercise judgement when managing online sources. As the amount of information produced daily continues to increase there is a danger that we will rely upon others to control and filter data for us. Information overload may cause physical and emotional distress decreasing one's ability to concentrate and remember. Consider using the following strategies to manage your information overload:

- *Develop organizational methods that work for you.* This might entail creating folders and placing items of interest into folders as soon as you receive them.

- *Do it now.* The first rule for improving efficiency is to act on every item the first time you see it, hear it, or read it.

- *Say "no" to junk mail.* Sorting through junk mail wastes time. Avoid junk mail by not having your name placed on mailing lists that do not interest you. Block e-mail addresses that you do not want. This can be done by using message rules in Microsoft Outlook Express or through the use of filters and anti-spam programs.

- *If you do not need or want it then delete it!* Keeping items that you have no use for contributes to clutter and can add to the feeling of being overwhelmed.

- *Stick to your focus.* When conducting a search remember your purpose. It is easy to follow other links that look interesting. This wastes time.

- *Try new search strategies and tools.* Stay with those that work well with you and abandon those that do not.

- *Restrict computer time.* Excessive time spent on the computer adds to stress, lowers work productivity, lengthens work days, and leaves less time for family and friends.

- *Avoid info-littering.* Be concise. Do not forward every e-mail that you receive to others. Do not send the same information via phone, Fax, e-mail, text and instant messaging.

Health Insurance Portability and Accountability Act (HIPAA) Compliance

The U.S. Health Insurance Portability and Accountability Act was passed into law by Congress in 1996. One of its major objectives is to ensure the security and privacy of health information. Other countries have similar laws or are working on similar legislation. HIPAA mandates administrative and technical procedures to protect the security and privacy of health information. These procedures include encryption of messages so that they cannot be read by accidental recipients, measures to guarantee the identity of the provider, restricting information provided to what is needed for treatment or billing purposes, and strict requirements for the storage and release of health information. Many patients and health care professionals use e-mail and the Internet to send, store, and process confidential health information. All health care providers need to be aware of HIPAA requirements. The U.S. Department of Health and Human Services provides extensive information on HIPAA regulations and their implications for health care professionals on their Web site *(http://aspe.hhs.gov/admnsimp/index.shtml)*.

An understanding of some of the issues surrounding use of the Internet will prepare you to use Internet resources wisely and efficiently. If you follow netiquette guidelines, you will be able to interact with others in a cooperative and effective manner. Knowledge of security concerns will help to protect computers from viruses, as well as protecting personal information and privacy. Thoughtful evaluation of Internet resources will aid you in making appropriate decisions about the information you discover.

CHAPTER

4

Educational Opportunities on the Internet

The flexibility of the Internet makes it particularly attractive for educational applications in health care programs, continuing education, consumer education, and the workplace. The Internet increases opportunities for informal and formal learning because it minimizes geographic and time constraints while it broadens the selection of offerings available to the user. Online resources are available to anyone with an Internet connection. Most resources, with the exception of live teleconferences, are available 24/7. The diversity of the Internet's offerings ensures that materials can be found to accommodate different individual learning styles and rates of learning. The text, video, and audio capabilities serve to reinforce learning. Links allow individuals to pursue material according to their interests or needs. The Internet also provides the means to disseminate information quickly before it becomes obsolete.

To realize these benefits, you must be comfortable with exploring online resources. Workshops, conferences, journals, and books about exploring the Internet help reduce anxieties and provide information about Web sites. Friends, professional associates, and librarians also serve as resource persons who can answer questions and guide you to sites of interest.

INSTRUCTIONAL APPLICATIONS OF INTERNET TECHNOLOGY

The Internet can support many forms of instruction, including online reference materials, computer-assisted instruction, tele-conferencing and Web conferences, multimedia presentations, virtual reality, and various forms of distance learning including Web-based instruction. The Internet nicely supports reference materials online eliminating the need to carry materials and providing access 24/7 from any location with an Internet connection. These materials include information on clinical guidelines, laboratory tests, drugs, medical conditions and treatment suggestions. E-books comprise one form of online reference materials that can be downloaded to a PDA or PC and updated as soon as revisions occur ensuring access to the latest information. Some ebooks are available free of cost but many of the traditional references used by students and health care professionals require a subscription. Most publishers have a separate section on their Web pages for ebook titles. Some other sites that provide links to ebook sites include *pdasupport.com, mobipocket. com, emedicine.com,* and *pdabooks.org"* With **computer-assisted instruction (CAI)**, interactive software is used to teach a subject. Advocates of CAI claim that it enhances computer literacy, aids in decision making, reduces computer anxiety, and improves reading habits. CAI also allows the learner to proceed at a comfortable pace, reduces learning time, and increases retention of learning.

The professional licensure examination review questions comprise a popular form of CAI from online. If you wish to view information about professional licensure examinations and review sample questions, simply enter a search with the name of the examination enclosed in quotation marks or parentheses. Sites focusing on these exams frequently belong to publishers of examination review books and companies. There are also sites that allow access to review questions with supporting rationale for responses for a fee.

Teleconferencing is the use of computers; audio and video equipment; telephone lines; and cable, satellite or network connections to provide interactive communication between two or more persons at two or more sites. In teleconferencing, learners at one site view and interact with an instructor and other learners at different locations. This allows educational organizations to establish collaborative programs, thus maximizing resources through shared classes and conferences. Teleconferencing is now available via the Internet. Although teleconferencing requires special equipment, home PCs easily may be configured for this capability. Webcams, or Web cameras, are relatively inexpensive cameras that can be mounted on or near the user's PC to capture his or her image and transmit it to other participants. Image and sound quality are determined, in part, by the speed of the connection. Teleconferencing via the Internet allows class content to be offered online along with assignments and feedback. This feature extends the reach of educational programs and continuing education courses to students who would otherwise be unable to attend sessions because of long commutes. Home desktop teleconferencing systems may not be suitable for the transmission of high-resolution images.

Web conferences, sometimes referred to as Web casts, are similar to teleconferences. Web conferences present content over the Internet. They may be live or pre-recorded. Presentation features can include slide show presentations, chat, live surveys, and white boarding, which is a technique that allows all participants see the same document at the same time and make changes that are visible to others. Web conferences eliminate the need for expensive travel. Web-based presentations can be viewed by persons who missed the original presentation. Pre-recorded presentations are less expensive than live versions, may be viewed multiple times, and may be used to generate income. Technical requirements are specified upon inquiry and registration so that users can determine in advance if they have the capability to view or participate in the conference. It may be necessary to change PC settings or download additional software.

Web conferences and Web casts are a popular means to present continuing education programs and business meetings.

Multimedia refers to presentations that combine text, voice or sound, images, and video, or hardware and software that can support these capabilities. The Internet supports multimedia effectively. Multimedia is an excellent medium for health care professionals because they must learn and communicate complex issues to clients. Research has shown that learning retention is facilitated with an approach that incorporates seeing, hearing, and doing. Group-paced instruction with multimedia decreases costs associated with individual instruction, increases comfort with computers, and improves learning as long as the environment is conducive to group use. One form of multimedia instruction that offers great promise is virtual reality. **Virtual reality** is a form of multimedia that fully envelops learners in an environment. It is already used to help medical students, surgeons, and other health care professionals with procedural skills such as, the insertion of intravenous needles and physical assessment. It offers the next best option to performing the skill on a real person but without risk to the learner or a patient.

Distance learning is the use of print, audio, video, computer, or teleconferencing capability to connect faculty and students who are based at a minimum of two different locations. Although it is available in other formats, teleconferencing via the Internet is one popular format for distance learning. Distance learning may occur in real, or synchronous, time, or via a delay. In real time all parties participate in the activity at the same time. With the delayed, or asynchronous, approach, the learner reviews material at a convenient time. The decision to use real versus delayed time influences instructional design, delivery, and interaction. Distance learning requires additional course preparation and organization by faculty and a concerted effort on the part of students to remain active participants. It can, however, be an effective means of instruction. Box 4–1 lists benefits for the student enrolled in a distance learning course. Distance learning may serve as a recruitment and retention mechanism for schools

Box 4–1	Benefits of Distance Learning and Web-Based Instruction

- Eliminates long commutes.
- Expands available educational offerings.
- May be available at home or in the workplace.
- Available 24 hours a day.
- Offers the opportunity to chat with the instructor or ask questions online.
- Eliminates geographic boundaries encouraging diversity in the student population.

of nursing and health care agencies because it may provide access to experts and cut costs. Distance education has become very popular, with many universities offering a full range of Web-based courses and programs. These courses generally employ a special type of software that provides a shell for faculty to present content, documents, and media. Common features include tracking mechanisms, threaded discussions, chat capability, a whiteboard, e-mail, the ability to post information and share files, administrative and security features, and the ability to test students online and keep an electronic grade book. These features provide a similar look and feel for online courses.

The Internet also allows you to perform online literature and database searches. Using a database allows you to efficiently locate content specific to your purpose. Online systems can search hundreds of thousands of databases in less than one minute. Databases contain standardized information pertaining to the items described. There are three main types of databases in libraries: 1) full text; 2) bibliographic; and numeric. Full text databases contain entire articles while bibliographic provide citations and abstracts only. Consider using numeric databases if you are looking for census information or similar statistics. There are thousands of different electronic databases covering a wide variety of topics. Successful database searches require some planning and a little practice. Box 4–2 provides tips to increase the success of your database search. Databases may be accessed through local libraries as well as Sigma Theta Tau's Virginia Henderson Library and the National Library of Medicine. The Cumulative Index to Nursing and Allied Health Literature (CINAHL), Medline, and PsychInfo represent the primary databases for use in health care. Users may also conduct searches outside of libraries although membership and fees may be re-

---

Box 4–2 Database Search Tips

- *Plan your search.* Identify your objectives then write out your topic in normal language first. Circle or underline individual concepts then identify possible variations. Determine what words and phrases are most important and how they are related. Consider all the words that should not appear. Determine the extent of information needed.

- *Choose the correct database.* Do some research on databases. Find the one(s) that cover(s) your subject then determine whether it covers scholarly or popular literature, the time period, what countries and languages it encompasses, and whether it provides access to full text articles. It may be necessary to use more than one database for a thorough search on your topic.

- *Learn how to access the database.* Determine the method to access the database from within the library as well as remotely either through library Web pages or independently. Many databases require subscription but are available through a library without an individual fee.

- *Become familiar with the features of the database.* Review and use the database vocabulary. It provides a consistent way to retrieve information that may use different terminology for the same concepts. Learn whether you can limit searches, use wild cards or truncation, and search by proximity and how to use these features. Limits restrict results by criteria such as dates, language, and type of publication. Wildcards or truncation employ an asterisk or question mark to stand for any character string to search for variations in key terms. Proximity provides meaningful context. In some cases terms are not meaningful unless they appear next to each other.

quired for other literature searches. There is no charge for a Medline search done through the National Library of Medicine. Increasingly, abstracts and full-text articles are available online, making it possible to locate and retrieve information quickly and at hours when libraries are normally closed. Information stored in many of these online databases are often inaccessible to the software spiders and crawlers that compile search-engine indexes and is sometimes referred to as the "Invisible" or "deep Web." It is several times larger than the visible Web.

- *Establish your search logic.* Use the Boolean operators AND, OR, and NOT for better results. "AND"-requires that all words joined by the operator be present to retrieve a record. The "OR" operator will retrieve any record listing either of the key terms. "NOT" eliminates items that you might expect to turn up in the search that you do not want.

- *Conduct your search.* Use advanced search screens whenever available because these are more powerful and precise than general screens. Place the most important words and phrases first. Search by field or subject rather than text or key word for more specific results. Check your spelling. Follow "more like this" leads when they appear useful. Use lower case when searching unless you have a specific strategy in mind.

- *Be systematic.* Each time you enter a database note name of database, date of search, and search paramaters used such as dates, terms and combinations, and hits to avoid repetition of effort. Use features that allow you to save or print this information.

- *Evaluate your results.* If results are too broad narrow the search by adding terms or limits. If results are too limited try using subject headings, variations in terms or other words that describe your topic. Learn how you can select, mark, print, save and/or e-mail specific records for future use.

- *Ask a librarian.* Librarians can help you to choose the best database for your needs and offer useful search tips. They can also help you request an inter-library loan for materials that are not available online or at your local library.

A number of Web sites also incorporate case studies as an instructional strategy. Case studies simulate situations found in clinical practice and are heavily favored as a good learning tool. One example of a Web site with links to case studies for various health care disciplines, including nursing, is Martindale's Health Science Guide at *http://www.martindalecenter.com.*

FORMAL EDUCATIONAL OPPORTUNITIES

Although a large portion of learning via the Internet has been informal, more and more formal offerings are now available. These take advantage of the reach extended by the Internet as well as its ability to provide interactive learning and incorporate multimedia. Some Web sites offer online continuing education, college courses, and even entire degree programs. Ideally, all health care professionals should develop the computer skills needed to access and use Internet resources. These skills may be integrated into basic educational programs and in continuing education.

Continuing Education

Internet courses offer a viable alternative for professionals who must meet their continuing education needs yet have limited funds and scheduling constraints. The Internet is available 24 hours a day to anyone with access to its resources. Furthermore, it can provide instant feedback and individualized instruction.

Many professional groups and private companies offer online continuing education. Web sites offering continuing education credits may be found through professional publications and organizations, as well as through searches. There are also sites that provide assistance with the development of educational programs. The Companion Web site at *www.prenhall. com/hebda* lists a sampling of sites that offer online continuing education.

Formal Courses and Programs

The proliferation of online courses and programs allows colleges and universities to recruit students from across the globe. Participants in these offerings are provided with a list of minimum hardware and software requirements. Courses may be presented live via teleconferencing or asynchronously. These courses and programs may be found through advertisements, mention in professional journals, word of mouth, or by a Web search. They are available at the associate, baccalaureate, graduate, and doctoral levels. Before you enroll in an online course for credit, however, investigate the offering to determine whether it meets your needs. Box 4–3 lists points to consider prior to enrolling in an online course or program.

Box 4–3	Online Program and Course Considerations

- Is the program or course offered by a recognized accredited college or university?
- Would it be accepted for transfer credit elsewhere?
- Has the program or course been offered online previously?
- What level of computer skills is required for class participation?
- What are the minimal hardware and software requirements? Look for courses and programs using proven technology to avoid technical problems.
- How do students participate in class?
- Is technical support readily available?
- Is the course or program entirely online?
- How have faculty been prepared to facilitate online instruction?
- What is the level of quality for customer service?
- Is specific information provided on curriculum and a timeline for graduation?
- Are graduates available who can talk with you about the course or program?

Health Care Consumer Education

Although many Internet resources are directed to health care professionals, other Web sites target the health care consumer. These sites may be maintained by health care institutions and professionals, government organizations, consumer groups, and even pharmaceutical companies. They commonly provide information about an organization or a physical condition or disease. In many cases they also offer online educational materials. Some sites allow consumers to ask questions and will provide answers within a specified time. Hospitals may include film clips of procedures and instruct health care consumers on how to prepare for specific diagnostic tests.

A growing number of consumers rely on the Internet for health care information. Information provided at these sites, however, should never be considered as a substitute for professional health care. Consumers should evaluate the credentials of the person or group providing information.

Evaluating the Educational Merits of Online Resources

It is important for the health care professional to consider both the quality of the information (as discussed in Chapter 3) and the instructional quality of online resources. These characteristics influence learning, and must be considered before recommending Web sites to others. Instructional design is important and should be considered after quality of information. As more health care consumers and professionals turn to online resources, it is important to select effective educational Web sites. Box 4–4 identifies some evaluation criteria that the health care professional should consider.

The Internet offers many educational resources for health care professionals and consumers. Successful use of Internet resources requires a level of comfort with the online world and the ability to locate and evaluate the quality of information pre-

Box 4–4 **Points to Consider When Evaluating Instructional Web Sites**

- Is it easy to locate?
- Are learning objectives stated and met?
- Is the material presented clearly?
- Is the content accurate and timely?
- Are links current and used effectively?
- Does the site allow individualized learning?
- Is feedback appropriate and immediate?
- Does the site use graphics, animation, and audio effectively?
- Is the author or sponsoring organization identified, along with contact information and credentials?

sented. There are a growing number of resources available to support students and faculty interested in online opportunities for learning. A partial list of these resources include several e-mail discussion groups and news groups, the International Centre for Distance Learning (*http://www-icdl.open.ac.uk*), the Canadian Association for Distance Education (*http://www. cade-aced.ca*), and the Journal of Library Services for Distance Education (*http://www.westga.edu/~library/jlsde*).

5

Research on the Internet

If you are interested in conducting research, start with the Internet. Using the Internet, you can research any topic from your home 24 hours a day. Some of the resources that you will find may have been available in other formats in the past, such as print. Other resources, including discussion groups, are only available electronically via the Internet.

IDENTIFICATION OF RESEARCH TOPICS

The Internet can be useful for all phases of a research project, including the initial identification of the research topic. Constant changes in health care and the health care delivery system make it difficult to keep up with the latest findings and to identify areas in need of further research. Online discussion groups and the publication of research findings help solve this problem. For example, the Nurseres listserv group, at *listserv@ listserv.kent.edu/archives/nurseres.html*, is a discussion list for nurse researchers. There are also discussion groups for specialty practice areas, education, and informatics. The Companion Web site at *www.prenhall.com/hebda* lists additional discussion groups that may be helpful in identifying potential research topics.

LITERATURE SEARCHES

Electronic databases allow users to conduct comprehensive literature searches over a shorter period of time than could be accomplished via a manual approach. A large number of universities and public libraries offer online databases for review. (In this instance online refers to databases that are available through Internet connections.) Many of these organizations require you to use an assigned user ID to authenticate your identity. The primary databases for searching nursing and health care literature are the Cumulative Index to Nursing and Allied Health Literature (CINAHL), Medline, and PsychInfo. These databases may be available in CD-ROM form or live via the Internet in libraries. You may also conduct literature searches on the Internet independently. Medline is available without charge via PubMed through the National Library of Medicine Web site. Individual users may access CINAHL and PsychInfo with a subscription. Each of these databases allows you to enter search subjects and then narrow the search by language, journal subset, and publication year. For example, you can limit a search to nursing journals or research reports. These features allow you to determine quickly whether research has been conducted in your area of interest and to review the reported findings. The user may view article abstracts online. Full-text article retrieval is available for many articles. Box 5–1 summarizes some advantages and disadvantages associated with online literature searches. Review Box 4–4 for ways to make your search a success.

ONLINE ACCESS TO DATABASES

The National Institutes of Health (NIH) offers access to several databases useful to nurses and health care professionals interested in research, health policy, and the identification of funded research projects. One of these databases, the Computer Retrieval of Information on Scientific Projects (CRISP), provides information on research grants supported by government agen-

Box 5-1 Pros and Cons of Online Literature Searches

Pros

- Searches may be completed quickly.
- Searches may be done without the aid of a librarian.
- Searches may be limited to specific years, languages, or journal subsets.
- Searches may be general or limited to request research reports.
- Online abstracts allow the researcher to determine quickly if a particular article suits his or her purpose.
- When available, full-text retrieval allows the researcher to obtain articles without searching for volumes on a shelf or waiting for copies to arrive from other sites.

Cons

- Searches require a basic level of comfort with computers.
- The person conducting the search must be able to narrow the topic area.
- Search results are directly related to the selection of search terms. Poor selection of terms may falsely indicate no or few articles on a given topic or provide an overwhelming number of articles of limited use.
- The researcher may need the services of a librarian to start the programs and to assist with search terms and limiters.
- Unless full-text retrieval is available, the researcher still must locate volumes and photocopy articles or wait for copies to arrive from other libraries.

---

cies. CRISP lists the following data for each project: title, grant number, abstract, principal investigator, thesaurus terms, and keywords. CRISP is available on the Web at *http://ott.od.nih.gov/TextOnly/crispdb1.html*. Search results may be printed or saved to disk. Several other agencies provide online databases useful to researchers. These include the following:

- The National Library of Medicine (NLM) at Web site *www.nlm.nih.gov.*

- The National Institute of Nursing Research at Web site *www.nih.gov/ninr.*
- Sigma Theta Tau's Virginia Henderson International Nursing Library (INL) at *http://www.stti.iupui.edu/VirginiaHendersonLibrary.* The INL provides information on nurse researchers, meeting proceedings, and access to databases that pertain to nursing research.

DATA COLLECTION TOOLS

Data collection tools may be located via online literature searches and discussion lists. The use of an existing data collection tool offers you the benefits of established validity and consistency, and the ability to begin research sooner without spending time devising and testing an instrument. A data collection tool is a device created to accumulate specific details in an organized fashion. Some examples include physical assessment forms, graphics records, and opinion questionnaires. Once a suitable tool is found, permission for its use often may be obtained more quickly through e-mail than through traditional mail. In the event that no suitable data collection tool is found, online resources can be used to help create and test a tool. Input can be solicited via e-mail, listservs, and Web sites on tool construction, specific items, and administration.

After the data collection instrument is selected, discussion lists may be used to solicit study participants and even as a means to collect data. E-mail interviews as well as surveys placed on Web pages may also be used to collect research data. It is also possible to develop online data collection tools. This will allow you to include features that may enhance the quality of information collected. For example, a participant who does not complete required fields receives a reminder message about this. The information collected can then be transferred into a database for analysis.

FUNDING SOURCES ON THE INTERNET

If you need to seek funding sources for research, various resources on the Internet may provide valuable information. Many of the agencies and groups that support research have a Web site that provides general information about the organization and possibly guidelines for seeking funding. It may be helpful to check the home pages of government agencies, such as the NIH, the National Institute of Nursing Research, the NLM, the Centers for Disease Control (CDC), the Department of Health and Human Services, the Federal Office of Rural Health Policy Funding Information, the Federal Register, the Agency for Health Care Policy and Research (AHRQ), and the Canadian Health Services Research Foundation. Research monies are also available for health care research from various foundations, such as the W. K. Kellogg Foundation and the Robert Wood Johnson Foundation. You may find other potential sources of funding by checking the Internet for the home pages of professional organizations, such as the American Nurses Foundation, Sigma Theta Tau, the American Nurses Association, or the Association of Women's Health, Obstetric and Neonatal Nurses (AWHONN). There are also databases, such as the Foundation Center and Grant Select, that list funding opportunities for health care disciplines. Finally, the home pages of foundations for specific diseases may provide relevant information. Examples include the Leukemia Foundation, the Skin Cancer Foundation, the Epilepsy Foundation, and the Myasthenia Gravis Foundation.

Use of the Internet can greatly support and enhance nearly every aspect of your research process. Internet resources, such as discussion groups, e-mail, and the World Wide Web, can provide you with ideas for potential research, research tools, literature searches, potential funding resources, and even specific tips for grant writing. In addition, use of these resources can provide the benefits of ease and convenience of access.

6

Career Resources on the Internet

JOB HUNTING IN THE 21ST CENTURY

The advent of computers and the Internet has revolutionized the job search process. Using the Internet can help you maximize your chances of finding a great job. Online job postings are available 24 hours a day, are more detailed than traditional classified ads, and provide a national and international reach. The Internet allows you to post résumés immediately and get virtually instant responses. For these reasons sending out a traditional résumé may no longer be enough to land an interview for the experienced nurse or recent graduate in the health care professions. The Internet and other computer technologies can help you research new job opportunities, get the attention of employers, and network with colleagues.

JOB SEARCHING ON THE INTERNET

The Internet can help you with your job search in several ways. Literally hundreds of sites on the World Wide Web contain classified ads. Most of these sites provide search engines so you can enter keywords describing the job you are seeking. Some examples of online career centers include *CareerBuilder.com*, *MedCareers.com*, and *Monster.com*. Looking through all the job listings on the Web can be very time consuming, so you may want to narrow your search to health care–related sites (see the Companion Web site at *www.prenhall.com/hebda*). You should learn about the features, functions, and services provided by the job posting Web site you are using. These often include services that match your posting to the existing job database and suggestions for writing résumés. Most sites have information about these services.

Another way to use the Internet in your job search is to post your résumé to a database. Again, it is probably best to choose a database that is specific to health care. One powerful way to use the Internet to help find a job may be less obvious: The Internet can be a great way to make contacts all over the United States. Interested in getting into home health care in Florida? There is bound to be someone out there, in a chat room or news group, who knows all about it. That person may even offer some suggestions on places that are hiring. Many people who spend time online are friendly and willing to help, so post your inquiry anywhere you think you may get a response. As always, be careful about divulging personal information. You can also use e-mail to network with contacts and stay in touch with former classmates, co-workers, and others who may be able to help you find a job.

The World Wide Web can be a great tool for researching careers and potential employers. Many hospitals and other employers have Web sites you can peruse. There are also Web sites for professional organizations, educational institutions, and other groups that may post useful information (see the Companion Web site at *www.prenhall.com/hebda*). Be inquisitive and creative.

HOW RÉSUMÉ DATABASES WORK

More and more employers are turning to automated applicant tracking systems to sort and track résumés. These systems are actually databases that allow prospective employers to use keywords to search for applicants who meet certain criteria, such as required skills, education, or geographic area. For example, say a health maintenance organization is looking for a pediatric acute care nurse. The employer enters words describing the ideal candidate into the automated applicant tracking system. In this case she may type in "pediatric," "acute care," and "registered nurse" as required keywords that résumés must include in order to come up in the search results. Other keywords for criteria that would be helpful for the job, but are not mandatory, may be included to further narrow the search. The tracking system then searches all the résumés in its system and retrieves those with the keywords the employer specified. Some tracking systems may display a list of résumé "titles" or header lines for each résumé retrieved, such as "LVN/home health care/Massachusetts." The employer can then select which résumés to see in full.

How do you find these résumé databases? Some employers have their own in-house automated tracking systems. Employers scan résumés received by mail into the system, and when a position opens up, they log onto the database to search for a candidate. Some employers are able to receive electronic applications via e-mail; these also are stored in the database.

Employers who do not have their own databases may use other generic applicant tracking systems on the Internet. Some of these databases encompass all job seekers in any field; others are geared to specific areas, such as health care. With these systems it is up to the job seekers to enter their résumés into the database.

There are several ways to post your résumé to an online database system, and techniques vary between systems. A common way is to type your résumé directly into the database at the Web site. Many systems allow you to paste your résumé from your word processor onto the database. You can often send your résumé via e-mail.

CREATING AND POSTING AN ELECTRONIC RÉSUMÉ

The electronic résumé has many things in common with the traditional résumé. Both prominently display your name, address, and phone number, and list your work experience, education, and special skills. However, there are several differences. Only prospective employers will see an electronic résumé if it contains the keywords for which the employers are searching. For this reason, many electronic résumés contain a keyword summary section toward the top, listing the standard phrases that describe the applicant's skills, areas of expertise, job titles, and credentials. It is a good idea to put the keywords in ascending order of importance. Using common abbreviations, synonyms, or acronyms for words used in the body of the résumé increases your odds of matching the employer's keyword specifications. For example, if you list "registered nurse" in the body of your résumé, use "RN" in the keyword summary. To determine what keywords to include in your résumé, look at the words used in the job listings and include those words that describe you. If you have access to electronic résumés, either on your home computer or at your library, you can see what keywords others have used as well. Both traditional and online résumés should be concise yet contain sufficient information to outline your qualifications, job history, and goals. Your main message and pitch should be relatively complete in the first five lines. If you have a number of things to say, summarize in the first few lines and go into detail in later sections. Use headings and lists to organize larger postings. Check your spelling, grammar, and punctuation. Use the spell check, edit for typos, and have someone else take a final look at your résumé if you are writing it with word processing software. A final version saved as text can be copied and pasted into online databases. Look for and use spell check features if composing your résumé on an online career center Web site for immediate posting.

Your electronic résumé may either be scanned into a computer or sent to a database via e-mail. The formatting you use must be readable in any system. Some kinds of formatting and typefaces will turn to gibberish or become unreadable in some systems. To make sure this does not happen, follow these rules of thumb:

- Choose a common typeface, such as Times Roman, Helvetica, or Palatino. Avoid fancy scripts, which are likely to degrade when scanned. Use 12- or 14-point type. Do not use graphics, shading, italics, underlining, or boldface. For emphasis, use capital letters sparingly.

- Use case appropriately. All lowercase is more difficult to read and looks as though you do not know how to use the shift key. Use title case for titles and sentence case for sentences.

- Avoid long paragraphs. Limit paragraphs to no more than four to six sentences or six to eight lines. Long paragraphs are hard to read.

- Use word wrap. This will avoid the appearance of awkward spacing in the finished product.

- Use standard keyboard symbols, such as asterisks for lists. Bullets often do not look the same once scanned or stored in a database.

- Eliminate page breaks and odd spacing. You want to ensure that your résumé looks like a single document.

- If you are sending your résumé electronically over the Internet, check whether there are any additional formatting specifications you must meet. Some databases require that you use certain margins or not use tabs. Many database systems require that résumés be sent in plain text or ASCII format.

- Examine your résumé before you send it electronically, by Fax, or postal service.

- If you are sending a hard copy of your résumé, print it using a laser printer. Be sure to send an original print, not a photocopy. If you must Fax it, use the fine setting.

- Use plain white 8 1/2 × 11″ paper with no folds or staples.

ISSUES TO CONSIDER

The advantage of getting your résumé into an automated applicant tracking system is that you will maximize your exposure to employers. There are, however, some disadvantages to consider.

It may be difficult for a recent graduate with little experience to shine in a database system because qualities such as independence, perseverance, and reliability are not usually entered as keywords in a search. If you are looking for your first job as a health care professional, you may not want to rely solely on an electronic résumé.

There are also confidentiality issues with database résumé systems. Although some systems restrict access to subscribers only, others do not. Either way, anyone, including your current boss (who could be a subscriber to the database you are using) can see your résumé posted there. Some services will provide users with a list of subscribers, but this is no guarantee that the information will not get back to your current employer. One way to help protect your privacy is to leave out identifying information about your current employer in your résumé. For example, you could write that you work at "a university medical center" instead of "The University of Texas Medical Center."

Before you post your résumé on any online system, review the site and the user guidelines. Is the site appealing and easy to use? Are there categories, such as profession, specialty, job type (full-time, part-time), and location, that facilitate the best match between your needs and the needs of potential employers? Use all available categories for your posting. Look for ads that supply information on salaries, bonuses, shift differentials, and other benefits. Review user guidelines for details about what formatting to use or avoid, how long your résumé will remain in the system, how to update your résumé, and the cost of posting your résumé to the database.

7

Internet Resources for Nurses and Health Care Professionals

This chapter provides an introduction to the diversity and wealth of information available on the Internet. A sampling of Internet resources of interest to health care professionals is provided here. The number and types of resources available on the Internet is growing explosively; therefore, it is not possible to provide an all-inclusive list at any one point in time. Because of the dynamic nature of the Internet, the following Web sites, listservs, and news groups may change, move to another URL, or cease to exist. In the event that one of the listed URLs yields a "not found" message, try a search as an alternative means to locate the site.

WORLD WIDE WEB SITES

Career Resources

American Mobile Healthcare
http://www.americanmobile.com
Travel staffing agency that offers temporary positions for health care professionals throughout the United States.

Association of Operating Nurses (AORN) Career Center
http://www.aorn.org/Careers/default.htm
The Web site of AORN, a professional organization, posts perioperative positions and allows online visitors to search for opportunities by geographic area.

CareerBuilder.com
http://www.careerbuilder.com
Database of help-wanted ads from across the United States; includes job search capabilities and employer profiles.

Cross Country TravCorps
http://www.crosscountrytravcorps.com/index.jsp
Travel staffing company for health care professionals.

Federal Jobs Net
http://www.federaljobs.net/employme.htm
Web site that provides information about job opportunities with the federal government.

Health Care Job Store
http://www.healthcarejobstore.com
Employment site for individuals and recruiters. Contains useful links to locate recruiters, research employers, conduct job searches, and manage one's own career.

HospitalNetwork.com
http://www.hospitalnetwork.com
Hospital Network contains news as well as links to product information and online catalogs, discussion forums, and career resources for health care personnel.

MedCareers.com
http://medcareers.com
Web site designed specifically to handle the nuances of the medical, nursing, and health care industry for job seekers and job posters.

MedConnect: Information Services for the Medical Community
http://www.medconnect.com
MedConnect Features interactive education, an interactive jobs line, updates on meetings and educational programs, and health information.

MediStaff
http://www.onwardhealthcare.com/index.aspx
MediStaff, a division of Onward Healthcare, is a job search service.

Monster.com

http://www.monster.com

A general career site for posting postions and resources.

Med Search

http://www.medsearch.com

National medical employment Web site with a résumé entry form and job listings. A division of Monster.com.

Pam Pohly's Net Guide

http://www.pohly.com/links.shtml

Web site containing links and reference materials for health care professionals and administrators for career enhancement, employment searches, and professional development.

General Health Care Resources

Cybernurse

http://www.cybernurse.com

Portal run by nurses that contains links to newsletters, continuing education credits, job opportunities, online shopping for books, as well as chats and a search capability.

Healthfinder

http://www.healthfinder.gov

Government Web site that focuses on reliable health and nutrition information.

Martindale's Health Science Guide

http://www.martindalecenter.com/HSGuide.html

Multidisciplinary, multimedia information resource that features links to many other valuable resources.

MD Advice.com

http://mdadvice.com/

This site provides health information, daily medical news, a health library, resources, drug information, articles, references, free medical questions and answers with experts, informative material, community support groups, live health chat, real-time interactive tools. It displays a seal from the Health on the Net Foundation.

Medical Matrix
http://www.medmatrix.org/reg/login.asp
Medical Matrix provides links to peer reviewed, indexed, and cataloged specialty and disease information.

Merck Manual
http://www.merck.com/mrkshared/mmanual/home.jsp
This searchable online reference provides information on various medical disorders and common treatment.

The Merck Veterinary Manual
http://www.merckvetmanual.com/mvm/index.jsp
This site serves as a comprehensive electronic reference for animal care information.

Nurseweek/Healthweek
http://www.nurseweek.com/index.asp
Online publication that provides news as well as links to continuing education and career resources.

Nursing Net
http://www.nursingnet.org
Popular Web site that features links, chat rooms, and message boards, and that provides a forum in which nurses can communicate with each other.

Virtual Hospital
http://www.vh.org
Virtual Hospital is a digital library for health care professionals provided as a public service by the University of Iowa. Its purpose is to make information that supports patient care accessible and to provide opportunities for distance education.

Web4Health
http://www.web4health.info/
Offers Free Online Medical Advice Answers providing more than 700 questions about psychology, mental health and relationships by a team of experts.

Resources for Nurses and Families

Association of Cancer Online Resources
http://www.acor.org
Provides credible information on cancer research and treatment.

Diabetes Mall
http://www.diabetesnet.com
Commercial Site that features articles and products geared specifically for the care and management of diabetes.

Resources for Nurses and Families
http://pegasus.cc.ucf.edu/~wink/home.html
Web site that provides a comprehensive list of links; maintained by Dr. Diane Wink from the University of Central Florida School of Nursing.

Nursetown.com
http://www.virtualnurse.com
Web site featuring job search capability, moderated specialty nursing chats, message boards, guestbooks, and conferencing.

The Virtual Nursing Center
http://www.martindalecenter.com/Nursing.html
Web site offering thousands of articles and links—a virtual plethora of information.

The Virtual Nursing College
http://www.langara.bc.ca/vnc
Online learning and teaching environment dedicated to the education and professional development of nurses with links to Medline, pharmacology resources, nursing terminology sites, job search sites, APA resources, hints on effective search strategy sites, and informatics resources.

Nursing Organizations and Associations

American Academy of Nurse Practitioners
http://www.aanp.org/default.asp
Web site that serves nurse practitioners of all specialties, providing conference information, information on certification, news, and links to relevant publications.

American Academy of Nursing
http://www.aannet.org
Professional organization that helps nursing leaders in education, management, practice, and research work with other health care leaders in addressing issues. "This Web site provides the following public information about the organization: history and composition of the organization;

mission; committee structure; its Living Legends, Honorary Fellows, and Scholar in Residence programs; and links to journals and educational offerings. It also provides services for members."

American Association of Colleges of Nursing
http://www.aacn.nche.edu
Web site that includes an interactive issues forum, institutional data and research, and career resources for nurses.

American Association of Critical Care Nurses (AACN)
http://www.aacn.org
The professional organization for critical care nurses.

American Association of Diabetes Educators
http://www.aadenet.org
Web site for the multidisciplinary professional organization dedicated to advancing the practice of diabetes self-management training and care.

American Association of Legal Nurse Consultants
http://www.aalnc.org
Provides a forum for education and exchange of information for registered nurses resulting within the legal field.

American Association of Neuroscience Nurses
http://www.aann.org
This Web site for this specialty organization contains links to news, publications, bulletin boards and online shopping members can also access the membership directions.

American Association of Nurse Anesthetists (AANA)
http://www.aana.com
The home page of the AANA includes client, professional, and member resources. Highlights include an Internet hotline and an Internet discussion list for certified registered nurse anesthetists (CRNAs).

American Association of Occupational Health Nurses
http://www.aaohn.org
Provides information about the organization and conferences, as well as access to the following services for members: career resources, discussions, and publications.

American College of Nurse–Midwives
http://www.acnm.org
Web site that serves as a resource to nurse–midwives through education, certification, and professional information.

American College of Nurse Practitioners
http://www.nurse.org/acnp
Specialty organization Web site that contains information about the group and its services.

American Forensic Nurses
http://www.amrn.com
Site dedicated to the dissemination of forensic information and education for nurses interested in and practicing in the field of forensic sciences.

American Holistic Nurses' Association (AHNA)
http://www.ahna.org/home/home.html
The AHNA Web site contains conference listings, chat rooms, and message boards for those interested in holistic nursing.

American Nurses Association/Nursing World
http://www.ana.org
Nursing World is the Web site of the American Nurses Association. Highlights include links to the Nurse's Career Center, the Online Journal of Issues in Nursing, the Credentialing Center, and an online book center.

American Nurses Credentialing Center
http://www.ana.org/ancc
Web site offering information about the criteria for certification for nurses practicing in a number of clinical settings.

The American Nursing Informatics Association
http://www.ania.org
Web site for nonprofit organization based in southern California that has members across the United States who share a common interest in informatics.

The American Nursing Diagnosis Association (NANDA) International
http://www.nanda.org
Web site for the organization committed to the development and classification

of nursing diagnoses for the purposes of contributing to the development of nursing knowledge.

American Psychiatric Nurses Association
http://www.apna.org
Web site that provides links to resources pertinent to the practice of psychiatric nursing and the advancement of mental health.

Association of Nurses in AIDS Care
http://www.anacnet.org
Nonprofit association's Web site that provides information about the organization as well as links to other sites of interest.

Association of Pediatric Oncology Nurses (APON)
http://www.apon.org
APON is the leading professional organization for registered nurses caring for children and adolescents with cancer. This site furnishes news as well as access to publications, education and membership services.

Association of Perioperative Registered Nurses
http://www.aorn.org
Provides links to career resources and education for nurses working in surgical settings.

Association of Rehabilitation Nurses
http://www.rehabnurse.org
Web site that offers information about certification, educational opportunities, and journals for this specialty.

Association of Women's Health, Obstetric and Neonatal Nurses
http://www.awhonn.org
Web site that features news releases, supports political advocacy for the health of women and newborn children, and provides opportunities for networking and information exchange via discussion forums.

Canadian Association of Critical Care Nurses
http://www.caccn.ca
Provides membership information and services as well as links to publications and pertinent research.

Canadian Nurses Association (CNA)
http://www.cna-nurses.ca
Web site that includes a calendar of events, links, publications, and more in English and French.

Center for Nursing Classification
http://www.nursing.uiowa.edu/centers/cncce
Organization established in 1995 to facilitate the ongoing research of the Nursing Interventions Classification (NIC) and the Nursing Outcomes Classification (NOC).

Emergency Nurses Association (ENA)
http://www.ena.org
The world's largest emergency nursing organization devoted entirely to the advancement of emergency nursing practice. Founded in 1970, the association has more than 24,500 members in more than 20 countries. Contains links to career resources, membership services, education, publications, research and scholarships.

HomeCare Online
http://www.nahc.org
Web site that provides membership information along with other resources for those interested in this specialty.

National Association of Neonatal Nurses (NANN)
http://www.nann.org
Web site featuring member information, conference schedules, and neonatology links.

National Association of Orthopaedic Nurses (NAON)
http://www.orthonurse.org
NAON's Web site shares information about the organization, certification criteria, awards offered by the group, as well as offering online continuing education.

National Association of School Nurses, Inc.
http://www.nasn.org
Web site dedicated exclusively for the professional organization of school nurses. It provides news, and links to HIPAA resources, position statements, surveys, and the NASN BookStore.

National Council of State Boards of Nursing, Inc. (NCSBN)
http://www.ncsbn.org
Official Web site for the NCSBN, developers of the National Council Licensure Examination for Registered Nurses Examination. It includes a database on acts and regulations, licensure requirements and maintenance, educational issues, multistate regulation information, and much more.

National Institute of Nursing Research (NINR)
http://www.nih.gov/ninr
The NINR is the nursing arm of the National Institutes of Health. Its Web site features research and clinical information for nurses.

National League for Nursing (NLN)
http://www.nln.org
The NLN is the resource center for nursing practice, education, and research. This site includes the latest information about NLN membership, constituent leagues, accreditation, testing services and tests, and meetings and workshops.

National Student Nurses Association (NSNA)
http://www.nsna.org
The NSNA is a national nonprofit organization open to all nursing students. Its Web site includes links to state chapters.

Oncology Nursing Society
http://www.ons.org
Web site for the professional organization of more than 30,000 registered nurses and other health care providers that contains links to news, educational opportunities, publications, research findings, and projects.

Sigma Theta Tau International Honor Society of Nursing
http://www.nursingsociety.org
The Web site of Sigma Theta Tau, the honor society of nursing, offers access to research materials, links, and information about the organization.

Wound, Ostomy, and Continence Nurses Society
http://www.wocn.org
Web site that promotes educational, clinical, and research opportunities to advance the practice and guide the delivery of expert health care to individuals with wounds, ostomies, and incontinence.

Other Health Care Organizations/Resources

American Academy of Child and Adolescent Psychiatry
http://www.aacap.org

American Academy of Family Physicians
http://www.aafp.org

American Academy of Pain Management
http://www.aapainmanage.org

American Academy of Pediatrics (AAP)
http://www.aap.org
The AAP is the professional organization "committed to the attainment of optimal physical, mental, and social health for all infants, children, adolescents, and young adults." This site provides services for members as well as a public side with links to new guidelines and recommendations, advice for parents, publications, and a list of practitioners by geographic area.

American Academy of Physician Assistants (AAPA)
http://www.aapa.org

American Academy of Professional Coders (AAPC)
http://www.aapc.com

American Association of Colleges of Osteopathic Medicine
http://www.aacom.org

American Association of Medical Billers (AAMB)
http://www.billers.com/aamb

American Association for Respiratory Care
http://www.aarc.org/index.html

American Chiropractic Association
http://www.amerchiro.org

American College of Clinical Pharmacology
http://www.accp1.org

American College of Physicians
http://www.acponline.org

American College of Radiology
http://www.acr.org/flash.html

American Dental Association
http://www.ada.org

American Hospital Association
http://www.aha.org/aha/hospitalconnect/sso/loginSuccess.jsp? action=INIT

American Medical Association (AMA)
http://www.ama-assn.org
The official AMA Web site contains information on medical science and education, advocacy and communication, and membership, as well as the AMA catalog and links to other medical sites.

American Medical Technologists
http://www.amt1.com

American Occupational Therapy Association
http://www.aota.org

American Osteopathic Association/American Osteopathic Information Association
http://www.aoa-net.org

American Podiatric Medical Association
http://www.apma.org

American Registry of Radiologic Technologists
http://www.arrt.org

American Society for Clinical Laboratory Science (ASCLS)
http://www.ascls.org

American Society for Histocompatibility & Immunogenetics (ASHI)
http://www.ashi-hla.org

American Society of Phlebotomy Technicians
http://www.aspt.org

American Speech–Language–Hearing Association
http://www.asha.org/default.htm

American Therapeutic Recreation Association
http://www.atra-tr.org/atra.htm

Association of American Medical Colleges
http://www.aamc.org

Canadian Association for Pastoral Practice and Education
http://www.cappe.org

Canadian Association of Speech–Language Pathologists and Audiologists
www.caslpa.ca

Center for Innovation in Health Information Systems
http://www.centerforinnovation.org/isi_dev.html
Web site committed to improving the health and well-being of individuals and communities through strategic application and management of information technology.

Clinical Laboratory Management Association
http://www.clma.org

Health Level 7 Organization
http://www.hl7.org
This Web site provides information about the HL7 standard, which is one of the standards governing the exchange of health care information between different information systems, as well as announcements of developments and upcoming conferences.

HIPAAdvisory
http://www.hipaadvisory.com
Web site that provides information on the Health Information Portability and Accountability Act (HIPAA) privacy, security, transactions and code sets, and national identifiers.

HIPAA.ORG
http://www.hipaa.com
Web site that provides a checklist to help you get started with HIPAA regulations.

Hospital Chaplains' Ministry of America, Inc.
http://www.hcmachaplains.org

International Society of Radiographers & Radiological Technologists
http://www.isrrt.org

National Healthcareer Association
http://www.nhanow.com

Professional Association of Health Care Office Management (PAHCOM)
http://www.pahcom.com

SNOMED International: The Systematized Nomenclature of Medicine
http://www.snomed.at
Web site for an organization committed to advancing excellence in patient care through the delivery of a dynamic and sustainable, scientifically validated terminology and infrastructure that enables clinicians, researchers, and patients to share health care knowledge worldwide, across clinical specialties and sites of care.

Accrediting/Regulatory Bodies

Canadian Council on Health Services Accreditation
http://www.cchsa.ca

Centers for Medicare & Medicaid Services
http://www.cms.hhs.gov
Web site of the federal agency that administers the Medicare, Medicaid, and Child Health Insurance Programs. Also contains information about the Health Information Portability and Accountability Act (HIPAA). The agency was formerly known as the Health Care Financing Administration.

COLA
http://www.cola.org
COLA is a nonprofit physician-directed, accrediting organization that promotes excellence in medicine and patient care through programs of voluntary education, achievement, and accreditation. COLA provides accredi-

tation to clinical laboratories. Its Web site provides news, a description of its accreditation and information services, online education, and links to membership services.

Commission on Accreditation of Rehabilitation Facilities
http://www.carf.org

Joint Commission on Accreditation of Healthcare Organizations (JCAHO)
http://www.jcaho.org
Web site for the nation's oldest and largest standards-setting and accrediting body in health care. It evaluates and accredits more than 15,000 health care organizations in the United States.

Continuing Education

CE-web
http://www.ce-web.com

KaplanCollege.com
http://www.kaplan.com
Provides online courses including some diploma and degree programs.

LearnWell
http://www.learnwell.org

Lippincott's NursingCenter.com
http://www.nursingcenter.com

Nursing Spectrum
http://www.nursingspectrum.com/ContinuingEducation

RnCeus.com
http://www.rnceus.com

SpringNet
http://www.springnet.com
Portal maintained by Lippincott, Williams and Wilkins providing links of interest to nurses, including some for job listings, career planning, conferences, continuing education, and an online bookstore.

Higher Education

All Nursing Schools
http://www.allnursingschools.com
Web site facilitating the easy location of information on any type of nursing program in the United States and Canada.

Association of American Medical Colleges (AAMC): List of Medical Schools of the U.S. and Canada
http://www.aamc.org/members/listings/msalphaae.htm

Association of American Veterinary Medical Colleges (AAVMC)
http://www.aavmc.org

Drug Information

CenterWatch, Clinical Trials Listing Service
http://www.centerwatch.com/main.htm
Web site featuring an international listing of clinical research trials and information about newly approved drugs.

CPOnline
http://www.cponline.gsm.com
The Clinical Pharmacology database is available online or for PDAs via subscription.

RxList—The Internet Drug Index
http://www.rxlist.com
Web site providing access to an online pharmacology database along with information on drugs, their interactions, and uses.

Government Agencies

Federal Trade Commission
http://www.ftc.gov/bcp/menu-health.htm
Provides diet, health, and fitness information for consumers and businesses.

FirstGov.gov for Seniors
http://www.firstgov.gov/Topics/Seniors.shtml
A portal designed to provide services for senior citizens inclusive of health, legal, retirement, tax and travel information.

Healthfinder®

http://www.healthfinder.gov/Scripts/SearchContext.asp?topic=375&page=2

Professes to provide access to reliable health information.

U.S. Department of Health and Human Services Indian Health Services

http://www.ihs.gov/MedicalPrograms/MCH/M/MCHdiscuss.asp.

Provides links to specialty listservs, as well as health and safety information.

Veterans' Health Education Library

http://www.health-evet.va.gov/healthinfo/Other_Links.asp?HideLeftMenu=Yes

Provides links to health information including benefits and services for veterans, special events and legislation, and a locator for VA facilities.

The Official U.S. Government Site for People with Medicare

http://www.medicare.gov/

Provides contacts, eligibility tools, information about prescription drug and other assistance programs, and the ability to compare dialysis and nursing home facilities

FoodSafety

Provides information on food safety, news and safety alerts, and advice for consumers.

http://www.foodsafety.gov/foodsafe.html

U.S. Food and Drug Administration: Center for Drug Evaluation and Research

http://www.fda.gov/cder/drug/default.htm

Provides consumers with drug information as well as news from clinical trials and newly approved drugs.

United States Department of Agriculture: Food Safety and Inspection Service

http://www.fsis.usda.gov/Food_Safety_Education/index.asp

Provides guidelines for food preparation as well as links to publications, frequently asked questions, and information on recalls.

United States Department of Health & Human Services
http://aspe.hhs.gov/admnsimp/index.shtml
Provides HIPAA information.

Computer Security Resource Center (CSRC)
http://csrc.nist.gov/virus/
Provides information on viruses, with links to news, vendors, and other resources.

CERT® Coordination Center
http://www.cert.org/
Center of Internet security expertise operated by Carnegie Mellory University and federally funded. Provides advisories, news and training to avoid matware and Web attacks.

Agency for Healthcare Research and Quality (AHRQ)
http://www.ahcpr.gov

Centers for Disease Control and Prevention (CDC)
http://www.cdc.gov

United States Department of Health & Human Services (DHHS)
http://www.os.dhhs.gov
The DHHS is the principal federal agency for protecting the health of all Americans and providing essential human services. Its Web page provides a wealth of information that addresses its programs, disease conditions, drugs, safety and wellness advice, policies and regulations, resource locators for health care providers and various facilities, as well as links to resources and publications."

United States Department of Health & Human Services, Grant Opportunities
http://www.os.dhhs.gov/grants/index.shtml
Web site that supports an online tool for finding and exchanging information about federal grant programs.

FirstGov.gov
http://www.firstgov.gov
Official Web portal for the U.S. government providing direct access to all government Web sites and information in one place.

U.S. Food and Drug Administration (FDA)
http://www.fda.gov/default.htm
The FDA is the federal agency that serves to protect consumers from unsafe products. Its site provides news, information about its services, an opportunity to report problems with products, comment on proposed regulations, and review job opportunities.

The Library of Congress
http://www.loc.gov
The Library of Congress Web site includes historical archives, legislative information, and a library service and research database.

Medline®: Access through the U.S. National Library of Medicine
http://www.nlm.nih.gov/databases/databases_medline.html
Web site that offers assistance searching in Medline.

National Institutes of Health (NIH)
http://www.nih.gov
The NIH Web site contains extensive health information, grants and contracts opportunities, and scientific resources.

National Library of Medicine: Extramural Programs
http://www.nlm.nih.gov/ep/extramural.html
Web site that includes information on grants and other assistance mechanisms.

Thomas, Legislative Information on the Internet
http://thomas.loc.gov/home/thomas.html
Web site that makes federal legislative information available to the public.

Unified Medical Language System®
http://www.nlm.nih.gov/pubs/factsheets/umls.html

The Visible Human Project®
http://www.nlm.nih.gov/research/visible/visible_human.html

Health Care Informatics

American Medical Informatics Association (AMIA)
http://www.amia.org
This Web site includes member information, links to special interest

working groups, conference information and publications, including the
Journal of AMIA.

AMIA: Nursing Informatics Working Group
http://www.amia.org/working/ni/main.html
This site provides information on the mission for this group as well as links
to resources, publications, and member services.

British Columbia Health Information Management Professionals' Society
http://www.bchimps.bc.ca

British Computer Society Nursing Specialist Group
http://www.bcsnsg.org.uk

Canada's Health Informatics Association
http://www.coachorg.com

Capital Area Roundtable on Informatics in Nursing (CARING)
http://www.caringonline.org

College of Healthcare Information Management Executives
http://www.cio-chime.org/default.html

Healthcare Information and Management Systems Society
http://www.himss.org/ASP/index.asp

Health Informatics Society of Australia Ltd.
http://www.hisa.org.au/

Maryland Society for Healthcare Information Systems Management
http://www.mshism.org

Midwest Alliance for Nursing Informatics
http://www.maninet.org/index.asp

Virtually Informatics Nursing
http://milkman.cac.psu.edu/~dxm12/vin.html
Web site designed to promote nursing informatics.

Online Publications

ADVANCE for Health Information Executives
http://www.advanceforhie.com

Advances in Nursing Science
http://www.nursingcenter.com/journals

Advances in Skin and Wound Care: The Journal for Prevention and Healing
http://www.nursingcenter.com/journals

AHANews.com
http://www.ahanews.com/ahanews/index.jsp
Online version of American Hospital Association News.

Amednews.com
http://www.ama-assn.org/amednews/index.htm
Online version of American Medical News.

American Family Physician®
http://www.aafp.org/afp.xml

American Journal of Nursing (AJN)
http://www.nursingcenter.com/journals

The American Journal of Maternal/Child Nursing (MCN)
http://www.nursingcenter.com/journals

American Nurses Association (ANA) Publications
http://nursingworld.org/rnindex/rnpubs.htm

Archives of Family Medicine
http://archfami.ama-assn.org

The Australian Electronic Journal of Nursing Education
http://www.scu.edu.au/schools/nhcp/aejne/aejnehp.htm

Australian Family Physician
http://www.racgp.org.au/publications/afp_online.asp

British Medical Journal
http://bmj.bmjjournals.com/index.dtl

Canadian Journal of Rural Medicine (CJRM)
http://www.cma.ca/index.cfm/ci_id/36550/la_id/1.htm

Cancer Nursing
http://www.nursingcenter.com/journals

Clinical Nurse Specialist: The Journal for Advanced Nursing Practice
http://www.nursingcenter.com/journals

Computers, Informatics, Nursing (CIN)
http://www.cinjournal.com
Journal designed to bring the sciences of computers, information, and nursing together while covering the application of computer technology to contemporary nursing practice. Print form of the journal is also available.

Critical Care Nursing Quarterly
http://www.nursingcenter.com/journals

Dimensions of Critical Care Nursing
http://www.nursingcenter.com/journals

Emerging Infectious Diseases
http://www.cdc.gov/ncidod/eid/index.htm
Peer-reviewed publication tracking and analyzing disease trends.

Family and Community Health
http://www.nursingcenter.com/journals

Family Medical Practice On-Line
http://www.priory.co.uk/fam.htm

Family Medicine Journal
http://stfm.org/fmhub/fmhub.html

Federal Register
http://www.access.gpo.gov/su_docs/aces/aces140.html

Gastroenterology Nursing
http://www.nursingcenter.com/journals

The Gene Letter
http://www.geneletter.org

Health Affairs
http://www.healthaffairs.org

Health Care Management Review
http://www.nursingcenter.com/journals

Health Facilities Management
http://www.hfmmagazine.com/hfmmagazine/index.jsp

Health Policy and Planning
http://heapol.oupjournals.org

Health Promotion International
http://heapro.oupjournals.org

Health Services & Outcomes Research Methodology
http://www.kluweronline.com/issn/1387-3741

HIV/AIDS Surveillance Report
http://www.cdc.gov/hiv/stats/hasrlink.htm

Holistic Nursing Practice
http://www.nursingcenter.com/journals

Home Healthcare Nurse
http://www.nursingcenter.com/journals

Infants and Young Children
http://www.nursingcenter.com/journals

Inside Healthcare Computing
http://www.insideinfo.com

JONA: Journal of Nursing Administration
http://www.nursingcenter.com/journals

JONA's Healthcare Law, Ethics, and Regulation
http://www.nursingcenter.com/journals

The Journal of Alternative and Complementary Medicine
http://puck.ingentaselect.com/vl=1476982/cl=71/nw=1/rpsv/catchword/mal/10755535/contp1-1.htm

Journal of Ambulatory Care Management
http://www.nursingcenter.com/journals

Journal of the American Cancer Institute: Cancer Spectrum
http://jncicancerspectrum.oupjournals.org

Journal of the American Medical Informatics Association
http://www.jamia.org

Journal of Cardiopulmonary Rehabilitation
http://www.nursingcenter.com/journals

Journal of Cardiovascular Nursing
http://www.nursingcenter.com/journals

Journal of Hospice and Palliative Nursing
http://www.nursingcenter.com/journals

Journal of Infusion Nursing
http://www.nursingcenter.com/journals

Journal of Medical Internet Research
http://jmir.org
Peer-reviewed transdisciplinary e-health journal that focuses on e-health, medical research, information, and communication on the Internet.

The Journal of Neonatal Nursing
http://www.neonatal-nursing.co.uk/default.lasso

Journal of Neuroscience Nursing
http://www.medscape.com/viewpublication/1065_index

The Journal for Nurses in Staff Development
http://www.nursingcenter.com/journals

Journal of Nursing Care Quality
http://www.nursingcenter.com/journals

Journal of Nursing Jocularity
http://www.jocularity.com

Journal of Perinatal and Neonatal Nursing
http://www.nursingcenter.com/journals

Journal of Public Health Management and Practice
http://www.nursingcenter.com/journals

Journal of Wound, Ostomy and Continence Nursing
http://www.nursingcenter.com/journals

Legal Eagle Eye Newsletter for the Nursing Profession
http://www.nursinglaw.com

Lippincott's Case Management
http://www.nursingcenter.com/journals

MedBioWorld
http://allnurses.com/jump.cgi?ID=237
List with links to online journals.

Modern Healthcare
http://www.modernhealthcare.com

Morbidity and Mortality Weekly Report
http://www.cdc.gov/mmwr

**National Cancer Institute Scientific Library
Online Journals**
http://www-library.ncifcrf.gov/onlinejournals1.asp
List with links to full-text online journals.

The New England Journal of Medicine
http://www.nejm.org
Web site offering the online version of the *New England Journal of Medicine*.

Nurse Educator
http://www.nursingcenter.com/journals

The Nurse Practitioner: The American Journal of Primary Health Care
http://www.nursingcenter.com/journals

Nursing
http://www.nursingcenter.com/journals

Nursing Administration Quarterly
http://www.nursingcenter.com/journals

Nursing Made Incredibly Easy!
http://www.nursingcenter.com/journals

Nursing Management
http://www.nursingcenter.com/journals

Nursing Research
http://www.nursingcenter.com/journals

Nursing Standard
http://www.nursing-standard.co.uk

Nutrition Today
http://www.nursingcenter.com/journals

Oncology Times
http://www.nursingcenter.com/journals

Online Journal of Issues in Nursing (OJIN)
http://nursingworld.org/ojin/index.htm

Online Journal of Knowledge Synthesis
http://www.stti.iupui.edu/VirginiaHendersonLibrary/OJKSNMenu.aspx

On-line Journal of Nursing Informatics
http://milkman.cac.psu.edu/~dxm12/OJNI.html

Orthopaedic Nursing
http://nursingworld.org/ojin/index.htm

Outcomes Management
http://www.nursingcenter.com/journals

PDA cortex: The Journal of Mobile Informatics
http://www.rnpalm.com
Web site for online journal that provides a wealth of information for persons interested in using mobile computing devices.

Plastic Surgical Nursing
http://www.nursingcenter.com/journals

Revolution—The Journal of Nurse Empowerment
http://ideanurse.com/advon

Topics in Emergency Medicine
http://www.nursingcenter.com/journals

The Weekly Epidemiological Record (WER)
http://www.who.int/wer

Other Online Resources

Cumulative Index to Nursing and Allied Health Information (CINAHL)
http://www.cinahl.com/

HighBeam eLibrary Research
http://www.highbeam.com/library/index.asp?

Publishers

Prentice Hall
http://vig.prenhall.com

Springhouse (SpringNet)
http://www.springnet.com

Search Tools

AltaVista
http://www.altavista.com

AskJeeves
http://www.ask.com

ClusterMed
http://vivisimo.com/clustermed

Copernic
http://www.copernic.com

Dogpile
http://www.dogpile.com

Excite
http://www.excite.com

Google
http://www.google.com

Highway61
http://www.highway61.com

Hotbot
http://www.hotbot.lycos.com

Ixquick
http://ixquick.com

Lycos
http://www.lycos.com

Medical World Search
http://www.mwsearch.com

Northern Light
http://www.northernlight.com

Open Directory Project
http://www.dmoz.org

Yahoo!
http://www.yahoo.com

Student Groups

American Medical Student Association
http://www.amsa.org

American Student Dental Association
http://www.dentalstudent.org

Other Health Care Sites of Interest

Academic Journal Directory of the University of Texas Medical Branch School of Nursing
http://www.son.utmb.edu/catalog/catalog.htm
Lists contact information for prospective authors for more than 400 clinical nursing, nursing education and research, and related health care journals.

AIDS Resource List
http://www.specialweb.com/aids

The Center for the Health Professions
http://www.futurehealth.ucsf.edu

FITNE
http://www.fitne.net
Web site that promotes the use of technology in health education.

Health on the Net Foundation
http://www.hon.ch/HONcode

MedConnect: Information Services for the Medical Community
http://www.medconnect.com
Web site that features interactive education, an interactive job line, updates on meetings and educational programs, and Health A to Z: A Search Engine for Health and Medicine.

World Health Organization
http://www.who.ch
Web site that features the world health report, the weekly epidemiological report, and the WHO newsletter.

Current Health Care News

CNN Interactive, Health Main Page
http://www.cnn.com/HEALTH
CNN's magazine-style site has a wide range of health care–related articles.

Data Interchange Standards Association
http://www.disa.org
Web site that contains information on electronic data interchange, links to conferences, and other standards organizations.

Electronic Healthcare Network Accreditation Commission (EHNAC)
http://www.ehnac.org
Web site for the nonprofit group that establishes standards for the electronic exchange of health care information.

Reuters Health Information Services
http://www.reutershealth.com
Reuters, the international news organization, gathers health-related information from a variety of sources. This Web site is an excellent resource.

Webopedia
http://www.webopaedia.com
Provides a quick reference to computer and Internet terms.

LISTSERVS

Nursing

Acute Care Nurse Practitioner Program Faculty (npacnp)
To subscribe, send an e-mail message to:
http://Majordomo@list.pitt.edu
In the body of the message, write only: subscribe npacnp

Hospice Care Discussion Group (HOSPIC-L)
To subscribe, send an e-mail message to:
http://LISTSERV.buffalo.edu
In the body of the message, write only: subscribe HOSPIC-L

Nursing Care Plans List (CAREPL-L)
To subscribe, send an e-mail message to:
http://listserv@listserv.acsu.buffalo.edu
In the body of the message, write only: subscribe CAREPL-L

Nursing Education (NRSINGED)
To subscribe, send an e-mail message to:
http://listserv@uvvm.uvic.cq
In the body of the message, write only: subscribe nrsinged

Nursing Informatics (NURSING-L)
To subscribe visit
http://mailman.amia.org/mailman
and follow the instructions provided.
In the body of the message. write only: subscribe NSGINF-L

pdasupport.com
http://pdasupport.com/
Site designed to help you find the best sources of support for your PDA with links to software, support, reviews, news, and other relevant information.

mobipocket.com
http://mobipocket.com/en/HomePage/default.asp
http://emedicine.com
http://pdabooks.org

Nursing Leadership (NUR340-L)
To subscribe, send an e-mail message to:
http://listserv@listserv.acsu.buffalo.edu
In the body of the message, write only: subscribe NUR340-L

Pediatric Nurse Practitioner (nppnp)
To subscribe, send an e-mail message to:
http://Majordomo@list.pitt.edu
In the body of the message, write only: subscribe nppnp

Perinatal Nursing (PNATALRN)
To subscribe, send an e-mail message to:
http://listserv@listserv.acsu.buffalo.edu
In the body of the message, write only: subscribe PNATALRN

Psychiatric Nursing

To subscribe, send an e-mail message to:
http://mailbase@mailbase.ac.uk
In the body of the message, write only: JYPC type "join psychiatric-nursing (First name Last name)" in the message field.

School Nurse Network (SCHLRN-L)

To subscribe, send an e-mail message to:
http://listserv@listserv.acsu.buffalo.edu
In the body of the message, write only: subscribe SCHLRN-L

Student Nurse (SNURSE-L)

To subscribe, send an e-mail message to:
http://listserv@listserv.acsu.buffalo.edu
In the body of the message, write only: subscribe SNURSE-L

Health Care

Biomedical Ethics (BIOMED-L)

To subscribe, send an e-mail message to:
http://listserv@listserv.nodak.edu
In the body of the message, write only: subscribe BIOMED-L

Health and Medical Informatics Digest (hmid)

To subscribe, send an e-mail message to:
http://Majordomo@maddog.fammed.wisc.edu
In the body of the message, write only: subscribe hmid

Home Health (HOMEHLTH)

To subscribe, send an e-mail message to:
http://listserv@list.iex.net
In the body of the message, write only: subscribe HOMEHLTH

Medical Libraries (MEDLIB-L)

To subscribe, send an e-mail message to:
http://listserv@listserv.acsu.buffalo.edu
In the body of the message, write only: subscribe MEDLIB-L

GLOBALRN

Provides discussion of issues relating to different cultures and health or health care and transcultural systems.
To subscribe send an e-mail to:
http://listsev@itssrv1.ucsf.edu
with the message: Sub GLOBALRN [your real name]

Venous (formerly IVTHERAPY-L)

Group for Intravenous Therapy (I. V.) Therapy Nurses.
To subscribe, send e-mail to:
http://majordomo@ohsu.edu
with the message: Subscribe venous

International TeleNurses Association (ITNA)

To subscribe send mail to:
http://listserv@listserv.bcm.tmc.edu
with the message: Subscribe itna [Your Name]

INFO-ALLIED-HEALTH

Discussion for librarians, and healthcare professionals which aims to identify and improve access to relevant sources of information, including library resources, for allied health professionals.
To subscribe visit
http://www.jiscmail.ac.uk/cgi-bin/webadmin?SUBED1-info-allied-health&A-1
and follow instructions provided.

Nicu_net

An international forum discussion of neonatal intensive care issues.
To subscribe, send an e-mail message to:
http://Listproc@u.washington.edu
In the message type, 'subscribe nicu-net (your name title).

Nursenet

An unmoderated, global electronic conference for the discussion of diverse nursing topics.
To subscribe, send an e-mail message to:
http://Listserv@listserv.utoronto.ca
In the message type, "sub nursenet (Your first name Your last name).

ProMed

Forum for the discussion of emerging infectious diseases, surveillance and response.
To subscribe, send a message to:
http://Majordomo@usa.healthnet.or
Type "subscribe promed" in the message.

AHRQ Nursing Listserv

Provides information about funding opportunities, conferences, and other nursing related activities.
To subscribe send a message to:
http://Listerv@list.ahrq.gov
Type, "Subscribe nursing listerv" (First name, Last name) in the body of the message.

ANPACC

Electronic discussion for advanced nursing practice in the areas of acute and critical care.
To subscribe send a message to:
http://ANPACC@yahoogroups.com

Camp Nursing (CampRN)

To subscribe send e-mail to:
http://Listproc@lisproc.wsu.edu
Type "Subscribe CampRN" (First name, Last name) in the body of the message.

Public Health (uhsph-1)

To subscribe, send an e-mail message to:
http://listproc@hawaii.edu
In the body of the message, write only: subscribe uhsph-1
YOUR FULL NAME

NEWS GROUPS

alt.abuse.recovery

alt.education.disabled

alt.health.ayurveda (ancient medicine in India)

alt.health.oxygen-therapy

alt.infertility

alt.med.allergy

alt.med.behavioral

alt.med.ems

alt.med.equipment

alt.med.fibromyalgia

alt.npractitioners

alt.psychology.help

alt.recovery

alt.support.abortion

alt.support.abuse-partners

alt.support.anxiety-panic

alt.support.arthritis

alt.support.asthma

alt.support.attn-deficit

alt.support.breast-implant

alt.support.cancer

alt.support.cerebral-palsy

alt.support.chronic-pain

alt.support.depression

alt.support.diabetes.kids

alt.support.eating-disord

alt.support.epilepsy

alt.support.food-allergies

alt.support.glaucoma

alt.support.grief

alt.support.headaches.migraine

alt.support.hearing-loss

alt.support.hemophilia

alt.support.herpes

alt.support.inter-cystitis

alt.support.kidney-failure

alt.support.menopause

alt.support.mult-sclerosis

alt.support.obesity

alt.support.ostomy

alt.support.prostate.prostatitis

alt.support.sinusitis

alt.support.skin-diseases.psoriasis

alt.support.spina-bifida

alt.support.stop-smoking

alt.support.stuttering

alt.support.thyroid

alt.support.tinnitus

alt.support.tourette

alt.support.trauma-ptsd

bionet.audiology

bionet.biology.cardiovascular

bit.listserv.autism

bit.listserv.blindnws

bit.listserv.deaf-l

bit.listserv.down-syn

bit.listserv.easi (computer access for people with disabilities)

bit.listserv.l-hcap

bit.listserv.medforum

bit.listserv.medlib-l

bit.listserv.snurse-l

bit.listserv.tbi-sprt (traumatic brain injuries)

bit.listserv.transplant

bit.med.resp-care.world

misc.emerg-services

misc.handicap

misc.health.aids

misc.health.alternative

misc.health.arthritis

misc.health.diabetes

misc.health.infertility

misc.health.therapy.occupational

misc.kids.health

misc.kids.pregnancy

sci.bio.microbiology

sci.bio.technology

sci.chem

sci.cognitive

sci.med

sci.med.aids

sci.med.dentistry

sci.med.diseases.cancer

sci.med.diseases.hepatitis

sci.med.diseases.lyme

sci.med.diseases.osteoporosis

sci.med.immunology

sci.med.informatics

sci.med.laboratory

sci.med.midwifery

sci.med.nursing

sci.med.nutrition

sci.med.pharmacy

sci.med.prostate.cancer

sci.med.psychobiology

sci.med.telemedicine

sci.med.vision

sci.psychology

sci.psychology.research

soc.support.depression.crisis

soc.support.depression.family

soc.support.depression.treatment

soc.support.pregnancy.loss

soc.support.transgendered

talk.politics.medicine (politics and health care)

Appendix A
Frequently Asked Questions (FAQ)

Q: I don't know much about computers. What is the best way to get started using the Internet and the World Wide Web?
A: There are a variety of resources to help you get started. These include
- A librarian
- A friend or co-worker
- Computer user groups
- Workshops or classes
- Books

Q: How can I find out about various types of Internet or Web resources?
A: Many potential sources of information exist. Some common resources include
- Journals and articles that list Web URLs related to specific topics
- Web links that lead you from one Web site to other related sites
- Performing a World Wide Web search using a search tool
- Other people such as friends, co-workers, and professional associates
- Advertisements

Q: What is a "hit"?
A: When you perform a Web search, the sites that are displayed by the search tool are known as *hits*.

Q: Do Web searches always yield a huge amount of useless information?
A: Because the Web contains an enormous amount of information, a general search can yield an extremely large number of

hits because every site that contains the search term is listed. When this happens, narrow your search criteria using the strategies outlined in Chapter 2.

Q: Why do I get different results when I submit the same search term(s)?
A: One possibility is that you may have used a different search tool. Each tool organizes the sites in a different way. Another reason may be that the search tool was updated between searches.

Q: Why can't I find a site even though I have the URL?
A: The address may be incorrect. Addresses must be entered exactly as listed, including spaces and punctuation and, in some instances, uppercase versus lowercase letters. Any variation will result in a failure to find the site. Even if you entered the address as it was provided, it may have been given incorrectly. Other reasons may include the fact that the address may have changed or is no longer maintained. An alternative strategy to locate this resource is to perform a Web search for the site.

Q: What is a bookmark?
A: You can use browser software to create a bookmark, which is a link to a specific Web site. This eliminates the need to re-member the URL and type it when you wish to revisit the site. Bookmarks can be saved to a hard drive or diskettes for reuse.

Q: Can I use bookmarks that were created with a different browser or computer?
A: Bookmarks typically can be used with different browsers or different computers. Occasionally problems arise when using different versions of software. In order to use bookmarks on an-other computer, you need to save them to a disk or save them to a file and e-mail them to a site that can be accessed from an-other computer.

Q: Why can't I access a site that I've been to before?
A: The site may be busy or the server may be temporarily out of order. Try again at a later time.

Q: Why do some sites take an extremely long time to load?
A: The site may be busy or contain a large number of graphics, or there may be a technical problem. Click the Stop, then the Reload or Refresh button to try again.

Q: Why is access to some sites denied to me?
A: Some sites restrict access for security and/or financial reasons. For example, some government sites only allow authorized users, whereas some commercial sites require registration and possibly a fee for access.

Q: Can I use materials that I found on the Web as references for my assignments or articles that I write?
A: Yes. Materials obtained from the Internet and Web can be acceptable references. However, consider the focus of the group supporting the site and the overall quality of the information. Students should first clarify this issue with faculty before submitting work that cites Internet resources. Some people are still not comfortable with this medium.

Q: What is the proper way to cite materials acquired from the Web?
A: Information obtained from the Web is subject to the same type of copyright considerations as other printed materials. This applies to all types of materials found on the Internet, including audio, video, and graphics, as well as text. A variety of styles are used in citing these sources. In general, the URL and the date of download must appear, as well as the title and author, if known. If specific formats for citation must be used, such as American Psychological Association (APA), refer to the appropriate manual or guidelines for examples.

Q: Can I get a computer virus when I use the Internet?
A: Although it is possible, prudent computing practices make this unlikely. Computer viruses are generally spread when files are downloaded and used without first scanning them for viruses. As long as you scan files prior to use and regularly update your antivirus software you should have few, if any, problems.

Q: Is it true that information is gathered about me whenever I visit some sites on the Web?
A: An increasing number of sites request demographic information and an e-mail address for screening and/or marketing purposes before the user is permitted to view additional pages. Look to see if the site has a stated policy about how information is used now, as well as any future plans for its use. If sensitive information is solicited, you may choose to exit the site without submitting it or check for the presence of information security measures, such as password protection and encryption, which is a process used to code messages. Unfortunately, unscrupulous parties may also collect and possibly misuse personal information. Use caution before you give out any information.

Q: What are cookies?
A: Cookies are tracking mechanisms that collect a limited amount of personal data about users. Originally designed to make access to favorite sites easier for users by eliminating the need to enter a password with each visit subsequent to the site, cookies also track popular links and provide information to programmers that will keep Web sites interesting to visitors. Web browsers use space on users' hard drives to store cookies. Cookies do *not* do any of the following:
- Harm the user's computer
- Obtain private information from hard drives
- Pass on information, such as e-mail addresses, unless specifically provided by the user
- Spread viruses

Q: What is spyware?

A: Spyware is software that secretly gathers information through the user's Internet connection, usually for advertising purposes, and sends it to someone else. It often comes bundled as a hidden component of freeware or shareware programs that are downloaded from the Internet. Spyware may also gather information about e-mail addresses, passwords, credit card numbers, and files. Spyware uses computer memory resources and bandwidth when it sends information back to the spyware's home base via the user's Internet connection which can cause system crashes and instability.

Q: What is spam?

A: Spam is unwanted or "junk" e-mail. It wastes time and clogs e-mail systems. It is used to spread advertisements and may be used as a vehicle to disseminate spyware. Efforts to curtail its growth include e-mail filters, legislation, and technical means. Avoid spam by not responding to online ads, setting up a "disposable e-mail" address, and not filling out online forms.

Q: What is spim?

A: Spim refers to unsolicited instant messages, often containing a link to a Web site that the spimmer is trying to market. Spim is spread by robots that harvest IM screen names off of the Internet and simulate a human user by sending spam to the screen names via an instant message.

Q: To what does the term "phishing" refer?

A: Phishing, pronounced "fishing," is the act of sending out e-mail that falsely claims to be from a legitimate enterprise in order to obtain private information that will be used for identity theft. The e-mail directs users to a bogus Web site where they are asked to update personal information, such as passwords and credit card, social security, and bank account numbers. The Web site is set up to steal information.

Q: How can I start a blog?

A: A blog is short for *Web log* which is a Web page that is used as a publicly accessible journal comprised of chronological entries. Once employed primarily by individuals for personal use, blogs have expanded to include news and research, a forum to communicate with employees and customers, a means to elicit feedback from employees, and even as a classroom tool. Blogs provide a voice for the "little person." The downside to blogs is that they can also be used to spread rumors, gossip, and speculation without accountability. Blogs may be found by word-of-mouth or through special search engines, such as *Feedster.com*. When starting a blog you should first determine what you want your blog to accomplish. Blogging software makes it easy to choose a template and start making entries. Blogs can also support video. You may opt to allow others to contribute to your blog.

Q: What is wi-fi?

A: Wi-fi refers to *wireless fidelity* and is used to refer to a protocol that allows wireless devices, such as notebook computers or personal digital assistants (PDAs), to communicate with other wi-fi devices through access points in public places, such as airports, cafes, and even parks.

Q: Why should I be concerned about cybercrime?

A: Cybercrime is growing rapidly as more people use computers and the Internet. Typically, it refers to using information such as social security, credit card, and bank PIN numbers stored or transmitted via computers to commit identity theft, access funds, or make unauthorized purchases. If you store or transmit such information on your computer or provide personal information on questionable sites, you risk becoming a victim. The lack of international laws makes it difficult to nearly impossible to prosecute perpetrators.

Appendix B
Exercises for Exploring the Internet

Exercise 1

The Nursing Computer Applications Committee at your hospital has been asked to evaluate whether Internet access on the clinical units would be beneficial. As a member of this committee, develop a report listing the potential uses of the Internet. Explain your rationale for each point.

Exercise 2

One of your clients has a rare genetic defect. The client is requesting additional information about his condition from you, but there are no reference books on the unit that address this condition. Develop strategies for how you might obtain this information using the Internet and electronic communication.

Exercise 3

You and your classmates in a community health nursing course are expected to conduct a health teaching project in a public high school. Identify and discuss Internet and electronic communication resources that you might use to gather material for this project.

Exercise 4

You have been asked to critique a consumer health care site. Identify the best features of the site as well as areas that might be improved. State why you believe the identified features are outstanding. Make specific suggestions for ways that the site can be improved.

Exercise 5

Identify measures that you should use for "safe surfing" of the Internet.

Exercise 6

You have been asked to help a colleague learn how to use a PDA to access reference materials stored locally as well as on the Internet and as a communication tool for instant messaging and e-mail. What major points should you address before your colleague starts to use his or her PDA?

Appendix C
Building Your Own Home Page

As part of the explosive popularity of the World Wide Web, many people now Web blog or design and maintain their own personal home pages. Many of these people use the home page as a tool to gain professional recognition or employment. This appendix offers basic resources and design consideration for creating your own home page.

GETTING STARTED

The best way to start your own home page is to plan it out. First, identify the purpose of your page. Identifying the purpose helps you to distinguish what information is appropriate to include on your page.

Next look at several home pages of other individuals. If you don't know where to find them, try visiting the Web site of a college or university. It is a common practice among faculty to maintain personal home pages. These pages can be found through links to specific programs or courses, or through a faculty directory. Review the pages you find and note what you like or dislike about each of them. You may also perform a library or Web search to determine factors such as the best screen and text colors to use and recommendations for font type and size to facilitate reading. You do not have to be a Web design expert to create a Web page that is visually appealing and conveys the desired information. Consider netiquette and good taste when designing your Web page, as others may judge you by the content.

Once you have determined the purpose of your home page, ask yourself the following questions as a guide to refining your plans and design:

- *How will I accomplish my purpose?* This question helps to pinpoint appropriate strategies for success. For example, it is appropriate for an individual seeking employment to place his or her résumé online. Examples of your work and links to references might be additional features. Detailed personal information, unless relevant to the potential employer, is not appropriate in this instance.

- *Where should I place and maintain my Web page?* Anyone with an Internet connection can create a Web document. ISPs can provide space for a home page that may be free or require an additional monthly fee. Other companies sell space as well, with varying monthly fees. There are even World Wide Web locations that offer free pages with some restrictions. Consider which service you would prefer to be associated with and the level of support that they offer. Next consider how much each service charges and whether you are willing or able to pay that amount.

- *What resources or tools do I need?* At one time it was necessary to have a mastery of the HyperText Markup Language (HTML) to design Web pages. Now most word processing applications offer the option of creating HTML documents. There are also Web authoring tools and Web sites that allow users with no knowledge of how HTML works to create effective Web pages by making a few simple selections. Web page authoring tools and sites that allow users to create their own Web pages can be located by conducting an Internet search, reviewing advertisements, or following the recommendations of others. You can also watch for free seminars or inexpensive workshops that may be offered at your school or workplace.

- *How long will it take to create my home page?* The actual time it takes to create a Web page will vary according to user expertise; content; use of graphics, video, and sound; and the inclusion of links to other sites. If these features are already in file format it is easier for the user to incorporate them into a Web page. Otherwise files must be created first. For example, images such as pictures or diagrams, can be turned into files using a scanner.

- *What type of technical support is available?* Schools and large employers frequently have support services available to provide assistance with the development of a home page.
- *How much time will be needed to maintain my home page?* It is frustrating to access Web pages and links that are clearly out-of-date. If the intent of your home page is to favorably impress others, it is necessary to invest time in its upkeep. The time required for this purpose will vary according to the nature of your pages.

PLACING YOUR PAGE ON THE WORLD WIDE WEB

Before placing your page on the Web, review it to make certain that information is correct, current, and without errors in spelling, grammar, or format. Test it to confirm that it works the way that you want it to. It is also helpful to include a date of origin or revision so that others may evaluate the currency of the information, and an e-mail or traditional address where inquiries can be sent.

You should request permission to use any copyrighted materials on your Web page. This includes just about anything that was not listed as "public domain," such as images, text written by others, and music. Failure to request permission prior to using copyright material may result in legal action.

GLOSSARY

Analog line A standard telephone line that transmits information using wave signals.

Antivirus software Set of computer programs capable of finding and eliminating viruses and other malicious programs from scanned diskettes, computers, and networks.

Blog Frequent chronological publication of personal thoughts and Web links; abbreviation for Web log.

Bounced e-mail E-mail that has been returned because of an inaccurate address.

Browser Software that accesses the World Wide Web and allows the user to move easily from site to site.

Bulletin board system (BBS) An online system that allows users to make announcements, share files, post questions, and conduct limited discussions.

Cable modem A popular alternative for high-speed Internet connections. These special modems use the same coaxial cable that cable television signals use and connect to a cable modem box, which is connected to an ethernet card in the PC.

Computer-assisted instruction (CAI) Interactive software used for teaching purposes.

Cookie A text file that is saved on your computer in a folder in your browser's directory; it stores information about the sites that you have visited as well as some information that you have entered in the site.

Cybercrime Commonly refers to the ability to steal personal information stored on computers, such as social security numbers.

Cyberspace The online world created by computer systems.

Dedicated telephone line A separate telephone line for use with the modem.

Digital line A newer type of telephone line that transmits information via pulse signals. This type of line is becoming common in business settings.

Digital subscriber line (DSL) Method for obtaining high-speed Internet connections that uses digital technology. This access also requires special equipment and an ISP.

Distance learning The use of print, audio, video, computer, or teleconferencing capabilities to connect faculty and students who are located at a minimum of two different locations.

Electronic mail (e-mail) The use of computers to transmit messages to one or more people in remote locations almost instantaneously.

Emoticons Symbols that are used in e-mail to express emotions or gestures.

Encryption A process that uses mathematical formulas to code messages.

File transfer The ability to move files from one location to another across the Internet.

File transfer protocol (FTP) A set of instructions that controls both the physical transfer of data across the network and its appearance on the receiving end. FTP is often used to transfer large files.

Firewall A type of gateway that is designed to protect private network resources.

Frequently asked questions (FAQ) Documents or files that introduce new users to a service, update new users on recent discussions, and eliminate repetition of questions.

Gateway A combination of hardware and software used to connect local area networks with larger networks.

Home page The first page seen at a particular Web location. The home page presents general information about a topic, person, or organization.

HyperText Markup Language (HTML) A popular language used to create Web pages. HTML provides special instructions for how text and graphics will be displayed, and how video and sound will be accessed.

Instant messaging (IM) An internet service that allows users to carry on a conversation in "real time."

Integrated services digital network (ISDN) One of the first high-speed options for Internet access. ISDN lines are about twice as fast as regular phone line connections, and they require special modems and other hardware.

Internet A network of many large and small computers and computer networks linked together so that they can communicate with each other. Although the Internet links government, universities, commercial institutions, and individual users, it is neither owned nor controlled by a single agency.

Internet relay chat (IRC) An Internet service that allows two or more users to carry on a conversation using typed responses in "real time." for the discussion of a specific topic.

Internet service provider (ISP) Company that run the computers and software, or computer programs, that enable access to the Internet.

Links Also known as hypertext, links are words or phrases distinguished from the remainder of the document through the use of underlining or a different text color. When a link is selected, it allows the user to move quickly to another Web page or document.

Listserv A type of e-mail subscription list or mailing list that copies and distributes e-mail messages to all subscribers.

Modem A piece of equipment that changes computer data into pulses or signals that can be transmitted over telephone lines, cable, or satellite.

Multimedia Presentations that combine text, video, and voice or sound, and the hardware and software that can support these formats.

Netiquette Netiquette is a set of informal rules that support etiquette, or basic courtesy to others on the Internet.

Search Engines Use automated programs that search the Web compiling a list of links to sites relevant to keywords supplied by the user.

News reader software Software that is needed by individual users to read messages posted on a news group. Many different news readers are available, and they usually come bundled with Web browsers.

Personal digital assistants (PDAs) Specialized hand-held devices used primarily to keep appointments, calendars, addresses, and telephone numbers.

Search meta tool Search tools that can shorten search time by employing several engines at once, often yielding more comprehensive data in less time.

Search indexes Software programs that help users find information on the Web by searching for pages or documents using keyword(s).

Spam Unwanted or "junk" mail.

Spyware Is software that collects data through the users' Internet connection without permission, and sends it to someone else.

Teleconferencing The use of computers, audio and video equipment, and telephone lines to provide interactive communication between two or more persons at two or more sites.

Spim Unsolicited IM, often containing a link to a Web site that the spimmer is trying to market.

Phishing Act of sending out e-mail that falsely claims to be from a legitimate enterprise in order to obtain private information that will be used for identity theft.

Trojan horse A destructive program that masquerades as a benign application.

Uniform resource locator (URL) A specific address assigned to a Web site that indicates the name of the document, as well as its Web location and the type of server on which it resides.

Usenet news groups Online user groups that provide a forum where any user can post messages for discussion and reply. Users do not subscribe to these groups, and they do not receive individual messages; users may participate at any time free of charge.

Virus A malicious program that can disrupt or destroy data, with effects that range from annoying to destructive.

Virtual Reality A form of multimedia that fully envelopes learners in an environment.

World Wide Web (Web or WWW) An information service that allows access to Internet resources. The Web features an easy-to-use graphical user interface (GUI) that supports text, images, and sound, as well as links to other documents.

Worm A virus that replicates, or makes copies of, itself. It may be passed to other computers in the form of a joke program or some other software program.

Wi-fi Refers to wireless fidelity and is used to refer to a protocal that allows wireless broad band another means of achieving connectivity to the Internet.

Index